# THE Special Diet Foreign Phrase BOOK

Your Passport to Healthy Dining in Mexico, Spain, Germany, France, and Italy

by Helen Saltz Jacobson

Edited by James W. Nechas

Translators: Lili Salinas Walsh (Spanish)
Karin Benthin (German)
Gaby C. Jacobus-Baudier (French)
Hugh Skubikowski (Italian)

Rodale Press, Emmaus, Pa.

**To the memory of Louis Vexler.**

Research Associate: Martha Capwell
Copy Editor: Dolores Plikaitis
Book Designer: Barbara Field
Project Assistant: John Pepper

Printed in the United States of America on recycled paper, containing a high percentage of de-inked fiber.

**Library of Congress Cataloging in Publication Data**

Jacobson, Helen Saltz.
    The special diet foreign phrase book.

        1. Food—Dictionaries—Polyglot. 2. Cookery—Dictionaries—Polyglot. 3. Diet—Dictionaries—Polyglot. 4. Dictionaries, Polyglot. I. Title.
TX350.J3 1982        641.5'63'03        82–11214
ISBN 0-87857-404-2    paperback

2   4   6   8   10   9   7   5   3   1    paperback

# Table of Contents

**Contents**

**Contents**

vi

**Contents**

# Acknowledgments

I am deeply grateful to the many cooks who helped bring this international stew to the table:

- Dr. and Mrs. Arthur C. Upton, who set the pot on the stove;
- Jim Nechas, my editor and the project's chef, who tasted and seasoned the concoction;
- Martha Capwell and Liz Wolbach, its *sous chefs* and fact checkers, who cleaned up after the chef;
- Barbara Field and John Pepper, the book's designer and her assistant, who planned the menu and set the table;
- Karin Benthin, Gaby C. Jacobus-Baudier, Hugh Skubikowski, and Lili Salinas Walsh, my translators, who garnished the stew with their knowledge of customs and cuisines from around the world;
- Emilia Bruce, who added special ingredients from Spain;
- Helen Soffer, my French typist and a consultant on many things;
- Professor Nicholas Marino, Suffolk County Community College, New York;
- Jack Lipkind, assistant head reference librarian, the State University of New York at Stony Brook, and his staff;
- Dr. Henry Masur, formerly Director of The International Health Care Service of The New York Hospital/Cornell Medical Center;
- Margaret Thieler, Senior Editor of *The Exporters' Encyclopedia;*
- Turner L. Oyloe, formerly Counselor for Agricultural Affairs at the American Embassy in Paris;
- Dr. David Albright of Brattleboro, Vermont;
- the U.S. State Department, which provided endless information through its health officers in American embassies in Spain, France, Italy, Germany, and Mexico;
- the hundreds of anonymous representatives of foreign governments who offered similar help;
- the cooperative restaurateurs in the major cities of our target countries who took time to answer our questionnaires;

- Gene, my husband, who tasted, listened, suggested, and encouraged no matter what shape the stew was in at the time;
- and lastly, the most savory spice in this international ragout: NECESSITY. There would be no book today if Gene and I had not spent years trying to explain our dietary problems to waiters and chefs around the world in chopped French, diced German, shredded Spanish, and minced Italian.

# Section One
# **Introduction**

Whether you are traveling for business or pleasure, your trip abroad should be a pleasant experience. But eating out in a foreign country can be an awful hassle unless you are bilingual or an expert at charades. And if you have a serious health problem that requires a special diet, these restaurants can be downright hazardous, and the peril and terror they excite may make you think twice about setting foot on territory where English isn't spoken. What you need, of course, is a special gadget, the science-fiction kind that would instantly convert your English into their foreign tongue, complete with a native's accent. Someday, when the present catches up with the future, you'll be able to buy this electronic mouthpiece, but for now, you'll have to settle for this very *different* phrase book. It's loaded with phrases that you can use to explain what you can or cannot eat in any situation you might encounter abroad and how you want your order prepared. If you can't pronounce the appropriate phrases, don't worry. All you have to do is point to them. Great, you say, but what happens after that? How do I understand a waiter's response? Simply show him the page where a number of possible replies to your question are printed. Not a word need pass between you: everything can be done by pointing to the proper words and phrases.

## **How the Book Is Organized**

It's divided into two parts. The first is full of tips, names, addresses, telephone numbers, and lots of other useful information for travelers headed for Mexico, Spain,

Germany, France, or Italy. This book won't tell you how to pack or dress, or when to put on a sweater against a chill, but it will tell you, very specifically, how to prepare yourself for health problems that might arise abroad. It will help you deal with all the niggling worries that can ruin a trip while it's still just a gleam in your eye.

If you follow the instructions in the first part of this book, your diet will be covered from the moment you board a plane or ship. There's also a letter about *your* diet that you can copy and send ahead to that quaint hotel where not a soul speaks English, not even the desk clerk. But they'll understand every word of this letter because we've translated an English model into Spanish, German, French, and Italian for you. If you wish, you can even compose your own letter in these languages by selecting phrases that best express your needs from a list we provide. What could be simpler? But be a sport: send it airmail or your letter may arrive long after you've returned home again. Oh, by the way: the letter does not require a response, but if you get one, take it to a school nearby and ask a teacher in the foreign language department to translate it for you.

The second part is divided into four different sections covering Mexico and Spain, Germany, France, and Italy. Although some of the information is geared to travel in these countries alone, most of the phrases will come in handy wherever Spanish, German, French, and Italian are spoken.

# Information from Other Sources

In each language portion of this book, you'll find extensive food lists, which describe common dishes and ingredients in the countries covered. But if you want even more details, you might want to pick up a book called "a menu reader." Here are a few pocket-sized editions:

**The Marling Menu-Master** series: menu readers for Spain, Germany, France, Italy. If your bookstore doesn't

have them, they can be ordered from the distributor:
Altarinda Books
13 Estates Drive
Orinda, CA 94563
Telephone: 415-254-3830
**European Menu Reader** (by Berlitz): 14 European languages in one book. If your bookstore doesn't have it, it can be ordered from:
Macmillan Publishing Corporation
Order Department
Front and Brown Streets
Riverside, NJ 08370
Telephone: 609-461-6500
**How to Eat (and Drink) Your Way through a French or Italian Menu** by James Beard. Try your bookstore or:
Atheneum Publishers
597 5th Avenue
New York, NY 10017
Telephone: 212-486-2700

## Health Books For Travelers

**Easy Going** by Mel London is a good companion volume to *The Special Diet Foreign Phrase Book.* It has a wide range of information: tips for travelers who have physical problems (cardiac patients, diabetics, etc.), for those who are deaf or blind, and for wheelchair travelers. If it is not available at your bookstore, it can be ordered from:
Rodale Press, Inc.
Organic Park
Department V. M.
Emmaus, PA 18049
Telephone: 215-967-5171
**Traveling Healthy** by Sheilah M. Hillman and Robert S. Hillman, M.D., is a guide to medical services in 23 countries. Try your bookstore or order from:
Viking-Penguin, Inc.
299 Murray Hill Parkway
East Rutherford, NJ 07073
Telephone: 212-755-4330

# The Wallet Card: A Shortcut to Using This Book

This little card will come in handy in the most tempting situations. Suppose you have left the hotel without your phrase book, intent on a quick return. But the road to hunger runs past these good intentions and through several happy and unhappy accidents. *Quick* has turned into four or five hours, and your stomach begins to talk to you. You pass a food vendor, and the delicious aroma of a dish on your "not permitted" list is speaking even louder than your stomach. You open your purse or wallet to make the purchase and notice your WALLET CARD. It reminds you of your diet. You tear yourself away from the vendor's goodies and dash to the nearest decent-looking restaurant. Without your phrase book, you can't read the menu to select exactly what you need, but—wait. . . . The waiter can read your WALLET CARD and help you find something that won't destroy your diet completely. The moral to this story is, of course, fill out the card now, and carry it with you at all times. You won't regret it.

Directions: Fill in the blanks on the FRONT of the card with appropriate words from the food lists found in each language section. PRINT LEGIBLY! A stranger you are asking for help *must* be able to read it. Show the FRONT of the card to your listener. Then open it, and point to both the questions and your respondent's possible replies. Be sure to show him the back of the card too.

# The Spanish Wallet Card

■ **I have a serious medical problem. I am not allowed to eat anything containing _____.**

Tengo un grave problema médico. No se me permite comer nada que contenga _____

_____

_____

_____

■ **Can you prepare my food in this special way?**

¿Le sería posible preparar mi comida de esta manera?

■ **Waiter/chef/manager: please point to your reply.**

Mesero (M),* Mozo (S)/chef/maitre: por favor señale usted su respuesta.

*fold here*

■ **No, I'm sorry.**

Perdone, pero no será posible.

■ **Yes, we can do it now.**

Sí, en un momento.

■ **Yes, but not today.**

Sí, pero hoy no.

■ **Starting tomorrow.**

Desde mañana.

■ **Wait, I'll find out.**

Espere, voy a preguntar.

■ **Return/phone at _____ o'clock on _____ (day) and we'll let you know.**

Vuelva/Hable a las _____ el _____(día) y le daremos la respuesta.

*(M) = Mexico; (S) = Spain

*cut out on dotted lines*

*fold here*

■ **Where can I find a restaurant that would cater to my special/ medical diet?**

¿En dónde puedo encontrar un restaurante que me pueda proveer con las comidas especiales requeridas por mi dieta médica/lespecial?

■ **Please PRINT the name/address/phone number.**

Por favor escriba en LETRA DE MOLDE el nombre/la dirección/el teléfono.

■ **Please show me on this map.**

Por favor enséñeme en este mapa.

■ **Please telephone for me. Thank you.**

Por favor, hable usted por teléfono de mi parte. Gracias.

■ **Please find the information for me in the telephone directory.**

Por favor, busque usted esta información en el directorio telefónico.

*fold here*

■ **I'll return at _____ o'clock for the information.**

Volveré a las _____ para que me dé usted la información.

■ **If you cannot help me, please let me speak to the chef/the manager.**

Si usted no me puede ayudar, por favor permítame hablar con el chef/el maitre.

■ **A mistake could have very grave consequences for me.**

Un error podría causarme graves daños.

■ **Thank you very much for your understanding and assistance.**

Muchas gracias por su asistencia.

# The German Wallet Card

- **I have a serious medical problem. I am not allowed to eat anything containing _____.**
  Ich habe ein ernstes Gesundheitsproblem. Ich darf nichts mit _____

  _____

  _____

  _____ essen.

- **Can you prepare my food in this special way?**
  Können Sie mein Essen auf diese besondere Art zubereiten?

- **Waiter/chef/manager: please point to your reply.**
  Herr Ober/Koch/Manager: bitte zeigen Sie auf die Antwort.

*fold here*

- **No, I'm sorry.**
  Nein, leider nicht.

- **Yes, we can do it now.**
  Ja, das geht.

- **Yes, but not today.**
  Ja, aber leider nicht heute.

- **Starting tomorrow.**
  Ab morgen.

- **Wait, I'll find out.**
  Einen Moment, ich erkundige mich.

- **Return/phone at _____ o'clock on _____ (day) and we'll let you know.**
  Kommen Sie/rufen Sie um _____ Uhr zurück, am _____ (Tag) und dann geben wir Ihnen Bescheid darüber.

German

Wallet Card

■ **Where can I find a restaurant that would cater to my special/
medical diet?**

Wo Könnte ich ein Restaurant finden, das Diät–Speisen zubereiten würde?

■ **Please PRINT the name/address/phone number.**

Bitte schreiben Sie mir den Namen/die Adresse/die Telefonnummer in *Druckschrift* auf.

■ **Please show me on this map.**

Bitte zeigen Sie es mir auf dieser Karte.

■ **Please telephone for me. Thank you.**

Bitte rufen Sie für mich an. Vielen Dank.

■ **Please find the information for me in the telephone directory.**

Bitte sehen Sie dies für mich im Telefonbuch nach.

*fold here*

■ **I'll return at _____ o'clock for the information.**

Ich komme um _____ Uhr zurück, um die Information abzuholen.

■ **If you cannot help me, please let me speak to the chef/the manager.**

Falls Sie mir nicht helfen können, lassen Sie mich bitte mit dem Koch/dem Manager sprechen.

■ **A mistake could have very grave consequences for me.**

Ein Versehen könnte schwere gesundheitliche Folgen für mich haben.

■ **Thank you very much for your understanding and assistance.**

Ich danke Ihnen für Ihr Verständnis und für Ihre freundliche Hilfe.

# The French Wallet Card

■ **I have a serious medical problem. I am not allowed to eat anything containing _____.**

J'ai un problème médical sérieux. Je ne dois rien manger qui contienne _____

_____

_____

_____.

■ **Can you prepare my food in this special way?**

Pourriez-vous me faire préparer quelque chose spécialement?

■ **Waiter/chef/manager: please point to your reply.**

Monsieur/Madame: s'il vous plaît indiquez-moi votre réponse.

*fold here*

■ **No, I'm sorry.**

Non, je regrette.

■ **Yes, we can do it now.**

Oui, nous pouvons le faire maintenant.

■ **Yes, but not today.**

Oui, mais pas aujourd'hui.

■ **Starting tomorrow.**

A partir de demain.

■ **Wait, I'll find out.**

Attendez, je vais demander.

■ **Return/phone at _____ o'clock on _____ (day) and we'll let you know.**

Revenez/téléphonez à _____ heures _____ (jour) et nous vous le ferons savoir.

■ **Where can I find a restaurant that would cater to my special/medical diet?**

Où pourrais-je trouver un établissement/restaurant, qui conviendrait à mon régime médical spécial?

■ **Please PRINT the name/address/phone number.**

S'il vous plaît, écrivez en caractères D'IMPRIMERIE le nom/l'adresse/le n° de téléphone.

■ **Please show me on this map.**

S'il vous plaît, montrez-moi sur cette carte.

■ **Please telephone for me. Thank you.**

S'il vous plaît, téléphonez pour moi. Merci beaucoup.

■ **Please find the information for me in the telephone directory.**

S'il vous plaît, cherchez-moi le renseignement sur l'annuaire de téléphone.

*fold here*

■ **I'll return at _____ o'clock for the information.**

Je reviendrai à _____ heures prendre le renseignement.

■ **If you cannot help me, please let me speak to the chef/the manager.**

Si vous ne pouvez pas m'aider, s'il vous plaît puis-je parler au chef/au directeur?

■ **A mistake could have very grave consequences for me.**

Une erreur pourrait avoir des conséquences graves pour moi.

■ **Thank you very much for your understanding and assistance.**

Merci infiniment de votre gentillesse. Votre aide m'est très précieuse.

*cut out on dotted lines*

*fold here*

# The Italian Wallet Card

■ **I have a serious medical problem. I am not allowed to eat anything containing _____.**

Ho un grave problema medico. Non posso mangiare niente che contenga _____

_____

_____

_____.

■ **Can you prepare my food in this special way?**

Può preparare il mio cibo in questo modo speciale?

■ **Waiter/chef/manager: please point to your reply.**

Cameriere/chef/direttore: per favore, indichi la sua risposta.

*fold here*

■ **No, I'm sorry.**

No, mi dispiace.

■ **Yes, we can do it now.**

Sí, possiamo farlo ora.

■ **Yes, but not today.**

Sí, ma non oggi.

■ **Starting tomorrow.**

Cominciando domani.

■ **Wait, I'll find out.**

Aspetti, mi informerò.

■ **Return/phone at _____ o'clock on _____ (day) and we'll let you know.**

Ritorni/telefoni a _____ _____ (giorno) e le faremo sapere.

Wallet Card

Italian

■ **Where can I find a restaurant that would cater to my special/ medical diet?**
Mi può dire dove posso trovare un ristorante che soddisfi le esigenze della mia dieta medica particolare?

■ **Please PRINT the name/address/phone number.**
Per favore, scriva IN STAMPATELLO il nome/indirizzo/ numero di telefono.

■ **Please show me on this map.**
Per favore, me lo indichi su questa cartina.

■ **Please telephone for me. Thank you.**
Per favore, telefoni per me. Grazie.

■ **Please find the information for me in the telephone directory.**
Per favore, mi trovi le informazioni nella guida telefonica.

*fold here*

■ **I'll return at _____ o'clock for the information.**
Ritornerò a _____per le informazioni.

■ **If you cannot help me, please let me speak to the chef/the manager.**
Se non mi può aiutare, per favore mi lasci parlare allo chef/al direttore.

■ **A mistake could have very grave consequences for me.**
Un errore può portarmi gravissime conseguenze.

■ **Thank you very much for your understanding and assistance.**
Grazie mille per la sua comprensione e il suo aiuto.

# Some Advice for Deaf Travelers

Fill in the blank space above the words "I have a serious medical problem" with this phrase:

I am deaf:   Spanish—Soy sordo (male);
soy sorda (female)
German—Ich bin taub.
French—Je suis sourd (male);
je suis sourde (female)
Italian—Sono sordo (male);
sono sorda (female)

Once you've filled in the card to your diet's specifications, tear it out of the book, trim the edges and fold the card along the lines indicated.

# Medical Tips

Before going abroad, there are certain things you can do to save worry about medical problems that might arise far away from home.

## What to Do before You Travel

**1.** Visit your physician well in advance of your departure. If you are taking any medication now, lay in an ample supply for your trip. But also remember to take a legibly printed prescription for the drug with you. This prescription form should contain the generic name of the drug plus the following information: the condition for which you are being treated, ALL the ingredients in the medication, and the strength of each ingredient. This information is important because drugs purchased abroad may have the same name but slightly different formulations and ingredient strengths.

**Caution:** Leave your medicines in their original, labeled containers. If you shift them to other containers, customs inspectors may confiscate them. If your medication is confiscated, however, don't despair. You can use the prescription form you've brought along to obtain a refill.

Another warning: Don't pack medications or prescription forms in your luggage; carry them on the plane with you. Then you'll have them if your bags find a different destination. One final precaution: The chances of your getting *turista* (traveler's diarrhea) or acid indigestion are practically nil, because you'll be sticking to your diet. But in case your companions eat and drink the wrong things, suggest that they ask their family doctor for an antidiarrhea medicine to take along. If acid indigestion can be a problem, your friends should have an antacid with them, one that is not nixed by a particular health problem. For example, if they follow a low-salt diet, their physician must choose an antacid without a heavy sodium content.

**Attention diabetics and other travelers on sugar-restricted diets:** Keep in mind that many antacids sold in the United States contain sugar as an "inactive ingredient." Often, this information is not included on the label, and several popular antacids contain 2,000 or more milligrams of sugar per tablet or per 15 milliliters of liquid. The same may be true abroad where some popular American brands are sold under similar or different names. If you think you may need an antacid, check with your physician before you leave. However, the *Physicians' Desk Reference* and other standard sources of drug information often do not list inactive ingredients, so you must ask your doctor to inquire for you.

**2.** Now, see your dentist. Give yourself plenty of time. There's no telling how much work you'll need done, and there won't be time for dental treatments while you're touring.

**3.** Do you wear glasses? Take an extra pair with you plus a copy of your prescription. Contact lenses? Carry an extra set and all the solutions you need for cleaning, sterilizing, and lubricating. Remember that many contact lens manufacturers recommend solutions specifically matched to their lenses, so bring your own brand along. They may not be available abroad. This brings us to the problem of lost contact lenses. Carrying a prescription with you may be no help, because most prescriptions contain the brand names of the lenses. If the optometrist you visit abroad stocks or can order your particular brand of contacts, you're in luck. Otherwise, you will need a new eye examination and a lens fitting, a proposition that usually takes several sessions.

**4.** If you have a serious medical problem, carry an identification card with you that describes your problem. For a nominal sum, the *Medic Alert Foundation* will supply such an identifying emblem, one that can be worn as a bracelet or necklace. Each medallion has a medical symbol engraved on one side while the other contains some brief information about your problem. The emblem also lists a U.S. telephone number from which more specific data about you can be obtained at *any* time. Applications for

*Medical Tips*

membership may be obtained from your physician or the nearest hospital. Or you may write to:

Medic Alert Foundation International
P.O. Box 1009
Turlock, CA 95380
Telephone: 209-668-3333 or toll-free: 800-344-3226
Important: Write well in advance of your departure. It takes time to transfer the data on your application to your emblem.

# Some Helpful Organizations

Ready, get set, go! You're off. You've said good-bye to your English-speaking physician, dentist, and optometrist. You're thousands of miles away from home. Did you check to see if your insurance policy would cover medical bills incurred abroad? What if you need to find a physician abroad and can't speak the language? Don't worry. Take two giant steps back and retrace a bit. Here's help: Take out membership in one of these organizations. Of course, you must be the final judge of which organization can help you most. This listing does not constitute an endorsement or recommendation of any of the groups. Request their literature and compare what they have to offer.

International SOS Assistance, Inc.
Two Neshaminy Interplex
Trevose, PA 19047
Telephone: 215-244-1500 or toll-free: 800-523-8930
   (outside Pennsylvania)
Members may call an SOS emergency number to obtain the names of qualified, English-speaking doctors or specialists in foreign countries. SOS can even provide emergency evacuation to the nearest facility capable of providing specialized care and, if necessary, arrange for a medically supervised trip back home.

Intermedic, Inc.
777 Third Avenue
New York, NY 10017
Telephone: 212-486-8974
Membership entitles you to a directory of English-speaking physicians in over 200 foreign cities.

Assist-Card Corporation of America
745 Fifth Avenue
New York, NY 10022
Telephone: 212-752-2788 or toll-free: 800-221-4564
  (outside New York)
Membership provides you with medical, legal, financial, and personal assistance abroad. It offers the services of multilingual doctors, dentists, attorneys, nurses, and other professionals. It also arranges ambulance or air transportation in emergencies.

International Association for Medical Assistance to
  Travelers (IAMAT)
736 Center Street
Lewiston, NY 14092
Telephone: 212-279-6465
A small donation brings you membership. Members receive a directory that lists the names of IAMAT centers in foreign cities. These centers will furnish you with a list of English-speaking physicians (internists and specialists) on 24-hour duty. The doctors come from a group located by IAMAT, and the list is updated annually. If you make an additional $25 donation, you can request a packet of World Climate Charts that outline weather conditions around the world and provide information on the sanitary condition of water, milk, and food in various areas.

The International Health Care Service (IHCS) at the
  New York Hospital-Cornell Medical Center
440 East 69th Street
New York, NY 10021
Telephone: 212-472-4284

If you live in the northeastern United States or plan to be in the New York area before your trip, you should make an appointment to visit the Center well in advance of your departure. The hospital staff offers pretravel counseling, physical examinations, immunizations, and posttravel screening. The IHCS also maintains an information system of English-speaking physicians and treatment facilities worldwide.

The IHCS concept is relatively new, but there may be a similar service at a large hospital or medical school near your home. Check. If you live in Canada, you can get similar pretravel counseling from the

Travel and Inoculation Service
University Clinics
Toronto General Hospital
John David Eaton Building
200 Elizabeth Street
Toronto, Ontario
Canada M5G 1L7
Telephone: 416-595-3670

Health Care Abroad (HCA), a Division of International Underwriters Brokers, Inc.
7653 Leesburg Pike
Falls Church, VA 22043
Upon presentation of the HCA card, medical services are provided for the traveler abroad. The HCA plan includes participation in the Medex network, which offers the traveler 24-hour-a-day doctor referral services, plus a directory of physicians and hospitals in the major cities of 128 countries. Each Medex-affiliated physician or hospital will accept the HCA card in payment for the services provided.

If you suddenly need to locate a qualified English-speaking doctor, phone the American embassy. If you are not in a capital city with an embassy, and you cannot find an American consulate (a sort of branch office of the embassy) or the consulate of another English-speaking country, you may phone the *nearest* American embassy or consulate and ask them to direct you to a U.S. government office closer by. You will find the telephone numbers and addresses of American embassies and consulates in each language portion of this book under *Medical Aid.*

# Before You Go. . .

There's something to the old line "If I knew you were coming, I'd have baked a cake." If hosts don't know they'll need a cake, they aren't apt to have one lying around. Do you, right now? Of course not. So, if you expect a culinary gesture upon arrival, you'd better call ahead. This precaution is especially important for people traveling on a medically required diet. If they expect a particular kind of cake to herald their entrance—one without sugar or fatty shortening or salt or whatever they can't eat—they'd better signal their intentions and expectations far in advance. Whether you're planning your own trip, working through a travel agent, or going with an escorted tour, get the names and addresses of the hotels you'll be stopping at and write them of your special needs. Here's a sample letter in English (and its translation into Spanish, German, French, and Italian) that you can send a hotel director before you go. Copy the translation, selecting appropriate phrases from the choices set off with slashes(/). Fill in the blanks with words and phrases selected from the "not permitted" list under your diet, your diet scenario, the basic food lists provided in *Part 2* of your language portion, and the food preparation appendixes. The sentence numbers in the English version of the letter match those in the translated models.

## The English Model

(1) Dear Director:
(2) I have reservations for _____.
(3) I plan to eat all my meals/most of my meals/some meals at the hotel.
(4) Unfortunately I have a medical problem and must observe a very special diet.
(5) I cannot eat anything containing _____.

19

(6) I would appreciate it very much if you would discuss my problem with the chef and arrange to omit _____ in the dishes served to me.

(7) For example, for breakfast I would like _____.

(8) The _____ should be _____ (method of preparation) and not contain any of the ingredients named above.

(9) For lunch/dinner I would like _____ or _____. (Copy sentence no. 8 for method of preparation.)

(10) I know you will understand my situation.

(11) I look forward to staying at your hotel and enjoying your country.

(12) Sincerely,

_____
your signature

## Spanish Translation

(1) A Quien Corresponda:

(2) Tengo reservaciones para el _____ (dates) de _____ (month).

(3) Pienso tomar todas mis comidas/casi todas mis comidas/algunas de mis comidas en el hotel.

(4) Desgraciadamente padezco de un estado de salud precaria y debo observar una dieta muy rígida.

(5) No se me permite tomar nada que contenga _____.

(6) Se lo agradecería mucho si pudiera explicarle el problema al chef para que se encargara de excluir _____ de los platillos que pediré.

(7) Por ejemplo, para el desayuno quisiera _____.

(8) El/La _____ debe ser _____ (method of preparation) y no puede contener ninguno de los ingredientes mencionados en la lista previa.

(9) Para la comida/la cena quisiera _____ o _____.

(10) Estoy seguro/segura que usted comprenderá mi estado de salud.

(11) Espero disfrutar mucho de mi estancia en su hotel. Agradeciéndole de ante mano su amabilidad y consideración.

(12) Atentamente,

_____
your signature

# German Translation

(1) Sehr geehrter Herr Direktor:

(2) Ich habe eine Vorbestellung bei Ihnen für _____.

(3) Ich habe vor, alle meine Mahlzeiten/die meisten meiner Mahlzeiten/einige Mahlzeiten im Hotel einzunehmen.

(4) Leider habe ich ein Gesundheitsproblem und muss mich an eine strikte Diät halten.

(5) Ich darf nichts mit _____ essen.

(6) Ich wäre Ihnen sehr dankbar, wenn Sie dieses Problem mit dem Koch besprächen und veranlassten, dass meine Speisen ohne _____ serviert werden.

(7) Zum Beispiel, zum Frühstück möchte ich _____.

(8) Der, Die, Das _____ sollte _____ (method of preparation) werden und keine der oben genannten Zutaten enthalten.

(9) Zum Mittagessen/Abendessen möchte ich _____ oder _____.

(10) Ich hoffe, Sie können meine Situation verstehen.

(11) Ich freue mich auf meinen Aufenthalt in Ihrem Hotel und in Deutschland.

(12) Mit freundlichen Grüssen,

_____

your signature

# French Translation

(1) Cher Monsieur:

(2) J'ai réservé du _____ (from) au _____ (to).

(3) Je pense prendre mes repas/la plupart de mes repas/ quelques repas à l'hôtel.

(4) Malheureusement j'ai un problème médical et dois suivre un régime très spécial.

(5) Je ne peux rien manger qui contienne _____.

(6) Je vous serais très reconnaissant(e)* si vous pouviez en parler au cuisinier et lui demander s'il lui serait possible de supprimer _____ dans les plats que vous me servirez.

*The e is a feminine ending, to be used by a female writer.

(7) Par exemple, pour le petit déjeuner j'aimerais _____.
(8) Le _____ devrait être _____ (method of preparation) et ne contenir aucun des ingrédients de la liste ci-dessus.
(9) Pour le déjeuner/dîner j'aimerais _____ ou _____.
(10) Je suis certain que vous comprendrez ma situation.
(11) J'espère avoir bientôt le plaisir de séjourner dans votre hôtel et de visiter votre pays.
(12) Veuillez agréer, Monsieur, mes salutations empressées.

_____
your signature

# Italian Translation

(1) Egregio direttore:
(2) Ho una prenotazione per _____.
(3) Intendo consumare tutti i pasti/la maggior parte dei pasti/alcuni pasti in albergo.
(4) Sfortunatamente, ho un problema medico e devo osservare una dieta speciale.
(5) Non posso mangiare niente che contenga _____.
(6) Le sarei grato se potesse discutere il mio problema con lo chef per stabilire di non usare _____ nei piatti da servirmi.
(7) Per esempio, a prima colazione vorrei _____.
(8) _____ dovrebbe essere _____ (method of preparation) e non deve contenere nessuno degli ingredienti sopraelencati.
(9) Per colazione/cena vorrei _____ oppure _____.
(10) Sono fiducioso di trovare in Lei comprensione per il mio problema medico.
(11) Mi auguro un piacevole soggiorno in Italia presso il Suo albergo.
(12) Cordiali saluti,

_____
your signature

# On the Way...

## Special Meals on Planes

Most airlines cater to special diets. If you give them sufficient notice, a custom-made tray will be put on board for you. Some airlines require only 24 hours' notice for certain diets, such as kosher, Moslem, and Hindu, but most require several days' notice for custom diets. Be safe: give at least 72 hours' notice and call your travel agent or the airline itself to make the arrangements. If you have a definite return date, be sure to make special meal arrangements for your return flight at the same time. Otherwise, you will have to do it at the other end where you may have language problems. Here are some of the diets that airlines accommodate:

- diabetic
- salt-free
- low-fat, low-cholesterol
- bland
- ulcer
- low-residue
- gluten-free
- vegetarian
- lacto-ovo vegetarian
- seafood
- baby food
- Chinese food
- kosher
- Moslem
- Hindu
- Feingold (hyperactive)

If your diet isn't listed here, that still doesn't mean it isn't available. Given enough notice, the airline's caterer may be able to provide it. The important thing is to call a reservations clerk well in advance of your trip and explain exactly what *your* diet requires. Most airlines will prepare almost any type of meal that a specific health or medical problem requires. So don't hesitate to ask.

# Special Meals on Ships

The chefs on cruise ships are old hands at dealing with requests for special diets. "Dieters," *Holiday Magazine* assures its readers, "need not hesitate. While many ships may specialize in a particular cuisine, their chefs pride themselves in serving whatever a passenger can dream up. And even though the stocking logistics are dazzling, special diets for passengers with medical or health needs can nearly always be arranged." Ask your travel agent to call well in advance of your departure to make sure the chef has plenty of time to get your special supplies aboard. When you make your request, be very specific. Write it all down *before* you speak with the agent. And remember, it's not enough to explain what you can't eat; tell him what you *can* eat. Bon voyage!

# How to Use the Diet Scenarios

In your language portion of the book, you'll find a series of diet scenarios. You are both star and director of these productions, and unknown waiters and chefs are your supporting cast. You can even be your own scriptwriter on this stage. Chuck out the lines that don't fit your case, and fill in the blanks with anything that's missing. Also highlight those lines you plan to use most often so you can find them when you're in a hurry. Fortunately, in *this* play you won't have to speak your lines. If you wish, you can simply point to them.

Although each scenario has been prepared for a specific diet, you can mix and match them. If you are on a diabetic diet, chances are your physician has put you on a low-fat, low-cholesterol diet too. If you have a cardiac problem, he may have prescribed a low-sugar routine in addition to the low-sodium and low-fat diets.

And don't forget: when you add items to the "not permitted" lists, PRINT LEGIBLY so they can be read easily. Go through the food lists in your language portion of the book to find the items you wish to add.

Here are the diet scenarios you will find:
• low-sodium (low-salt) diet
• diabetic (low-sugar) diet
• low-fat, low-cholesterol diet
• ulcer, bland, soft, and low-residue diet
• custom-made diet

If you have a dietary need not covered in any of the scenarios, the *last* scenario in your language portion of the book is just for you. We have prepared phrases and sentences that you can use to fashion your own, tailor-made script. You'll have to scavenge here and there, choosing items from the food lists, borrowing bits and pieces from other diet scenarios, but you can design a model that suits your specific needs. For instance, even patients on kidney dialysis are traveling now and arranging for regular treatments at dialysis centers throughout the world. If you're one of them, start with the low-sodium scenario. Then, select low-potassium and low-protein foods from the food lists, and use the food preparation appendixes to be sure your foods and beverages are properly prepared. If you're planning to drink bottled water, use the table on the opposite page to check its sodium and potassium content.

# A Note on Drinking Bottled Water in a Foreign Country

If you are on a sodium- or potassium-restricted diet, keep this table handy when you order bottled water. Remember, of course, that the mineral content of almost anything varies from sample to sample and even from test to test. So use this table as a comparative guide only. Sometimes a water's mineral content will also appear on the bottle, either on a paper label or printed directly on the glass. To evaluate this information use the following guide. The international chemical symbols are:

potassium—K
sodium—Na

Or look for the whole word, as shown here:

| | | |
|---|---|---|
| Spanish | sodio | potasio |
| German | Sodium (Natrium) | Potassium |
| French | sodium | potassium |
| Italian | sodio | potassio |

If a chemical analysis appears on the bottle, it usually lists substances in milligrams per liter of water. A liter is roughly equivalent to a quart. Sometimes the analysis is listed in grams per liter. To convert grams to milligrams, move the decimal point three places to the right. For example, if the sodium (Na) content is shown as 0.0069 grams per liter, moving the decimal point three places to the right gives you 6.9 milligrams per liter.

And now the bottled waters:

## Sodium and Potassium Content in Bottled Waters

| Water (1 liter) | Sodium (milligrams) | Potassium (milligrams) |
|---|---|---|
| Spa | 2.9 | 0.6 |
| Vittel | 4.7 | 3.3 |
| Fiuggi | 6.8 | 4.0 |
| Evian | 6.9 | 2.3 |
| Contrexeville | 9.0 | 3.0 |
| Perrier | 14.5 | 1.0 |
| San Pellegrino | 44.2 | 4.2 |
| Solares | 92.1 | 0.3 |
| Badoit | 205.0 | 16.0 |
| Peñafiel | 309.9 | 19.0 |
| Apollinaris | 630.5 | 33.6 |
| Vichy Celestins | 1223.0 | 75.4 |
| Vichy Saint-Yorre | 1676.0 | 105.0 |

**Note:** Evian and Vittel, low in sodium and potassium, are sold in Spain, Germany, and France; Fiuggi is sold in Italy; Peñafiel comes from Mexico.

# Section Two:
# Say It
# in
# Spanish

# Spanish Pronunciation

The sound patterns in Spanish are fairly regular, and so its pronunciation is relatively easy—once you've discovered which vowel sounds are different from English, which consonants are unlike our own, and how Spanish speakers tend to accent their syllables.

## Vowels

**A**   as in FATHER: *mamá*
**E**   as in ELLEN: *estar*
**I**   as in MACHINE: *día*
**O**   as in OVER: *como*
**U**   as in RUMOR: *usted*

## Consonants

**B** and **V**   both pronounced like BOY: *bebé, vaca*
**CH**   as in CHILDREN: *leche*
**LL**   as in YES: *lluvia*
**QU**   as in CAKE, the U is silent: *queso*
**Z** and **C**   before E or I pronounced like the **S** in SALLY: *zero, Cecilia*
**C**   before all other letters pronounced as in CAT: *cantar*
**Ñ**   as in the **NI** of ONION: *niño*
**J**   as if you exaggerated the H in HELLO: *jefe*
**G**   before E and I is also like an exaggerated H: *Virginia*
**GUI/GUE**   as in GUESS: *Guillermo, guerra*
**GUA/GUO**   the G is pronounced as in GOAT, but this time the U is also pronounced: *agua, antiguo*
**H**   the H is always silent: *hermana*
*The pronunciation of all other consonants is close to the English pronunciation.*

30

# Accentuation and Syllables

**1.** The accent marks found in such words as *mamá* and *acción* specify that you should stress the marked syllable. Thus, in Spanish, *mamá* would be stressed *ma-MÁ, acción, ac-CIÓN.*

**2.** Words that end in a vowel or in the consonants N or S are stressed on the next to the last syllable: *casas* is *CA-sas, señora, se-ÑO-ra.*

**3.** Words that end in a consonant, except for N or S, are stressed on the last syllable: *libertad* is *li-ber-TAD, español, es-pa-ÑOL.*

**4.** Any exceptions to these rules have a written accent on the stressed syllable: *tradición* is *tra-di-CIÓN; inglés, in-GLÉS, aquí, a-QUÍ.*

# Basic Expressions in Spanish

- **Yes**
  Sí

- **No**
  No

- **Hello (a familiar form, used only among friends)**
  ¡Hola!

- **Please**
  Por favor

- **Thank you**
  Gracias

- **Excuse me**
  Discúlpeme

- **Pardon me**
  Perdone usted

- **Good morning, Good afternoon, Good evening**
  Buenos días, Buenas tardas, Buenas noches

- **Good night, Good-bye**
  Buenas noches, Hasta luego

- **Where is the ladies'/men's room?**
  ¿Dónde está el baño para damas/caballeros?

■ **My name is Mr./Mrs./Miss _____.**
Soy el señor/la señora/la señorita _____.

■ **I am staying at _____.**
Estoy hospedado en _____.

■ **Can you help me?**
¿Podría usted asistirme?

■ **Do you speak English?**
¿Habla usted inglés?

■ **Does anyone here speak English?**
¿Hay álguien aquí que hable inglés?

■ **Can you find anyone who speaks English?**
¿Podría usted buscar a álguien que hable inglés?

■ **I do not understand.**
No comprendo.

■ **Please speak slowly.**
Por favor hable usted más despacio.

■ **Please repeat it.**
Por favor repita su respuesta.

■ **Please PRINT the directions.**
Por favor escriba las direcciones en LETRA DE MOLDE.

■ **Please PRINT it.**
Por favor escríbalo en LETRA DE MOLDE.

■ **Please PRINT the name, address, and telephone number.**
Por favor escriba en LETRA DE MOLDE el nombre, la dirección, y el teléfono.

- **Please show me on this map.**
  Por favor enséñeme en el mapa.

- **Please show me on this map where I am.**
  Por favor enséñeme en este mapa en dónde estoy.

- **Please draw a map/sketch for me.**
  Por favor hágame un mapa/un dibujo.

- **Please call this number for me. Thank you.**
  Hágame usted el favor de hablar por teléfono a este número. Gracias.

- **Where is the nearest _____?**
  ¿Dónde está _____ más cercano/a?
  - **hospital/clinic**
    el hospital/la clínica
  - **first aid facility**
    la clínica de primeros auxilios
  - **diet/health food/natural food restaurant**
    el restaurante naturista/dietético

- **Is the restaurant open/closed now?**
  ¿El restaurante, está abierto/cerrado ahora?

- **Please point to the days and hours it is open/closed.**
  Por favor enséñeme los días y las horas en que está abierto/cerrado.

- **Monday**
  lunes

- **Tuesday**
  martes

- **Wednesday**
  miércoles

- **Thursday**
  jueves

- **Friday**
  viernes

- **Saturday**
  sábado

- **Sunday**
  domingo

- **a quarter past**
  y cuarto

- **half past**
  y media

- **a quarter to**
  menos cuarto

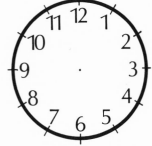

- **A.M.**
  de la mañana

- **P.M.**
  de la tarde

- **How much is this? Please write it down. (For a list of numbers, see page 100.)**
  ¿Cuánto cuesta esto? Por favor escríbalo.

- **Do you have _____?**
  ¿Tiene usted _____?

- **I would like _____.**
  Quisiera _____.

- **Please give me _____.**
  Por favor, déme _____.

# Water, Food, and Drink in Mexico and Spain-Some Precautions

## Mexico

You can walk in it, swim in it, even wash your face with it, but don't drink the tap water here or brush your teeth with it. Of course, we're not suggesting that you leave either your teeth or your toothbrush at home. Take both with you and use bottled water for the cleanup. Sure, it's not the cheapest way to get the job done, but if you balance the expense against the emotional and physical cost of a case of intestinal distress, you won't mind shelling out a few pesos for safe water.

Yes, there *are* ways of making Mexican tap water safe for drinking. It can be boiled for ten minutes or *more*, and then stored in the *same* pot or in another *sterilized* container. An alternative to boiling is the use of a chemical sterilizing agent. Any one of the following will work: Halazone tablets, Potable Aqua (sometimes called Pota Aqua) pills, or a small bottle of iodine. But remember—boiling is the safest method: Halazone, the most common of the special chemicals, has a shelf life of just six months and is only effective against certain bacteria. Still, the chemicals are reasonably safe. To use iodine, add five drops of tincture of iodine to each quart of water and allow it to act for 30 minutes. Follow package directions for the chemical agents, but be sure to double the number of tablets for cloudy, dirty, or discolored water. Halazone and

37

Potable Aqua can be purchased in the United States at pharmacies and camping supply stores. If you can't find either, ask your pharmacist to order Halazone tablets from:
Abbott Laboratories
14th Street and Sheridan Road
North Chicago, IL 60064
Potable Aqua can be ordered from:
Wisconsin Pharmacal Co.
2535 South 170th Street
New Berlin, WI 53151

The safest and easiest thing to do when traveling in Mexico is to use bottled water and avoid tap water entirely. However, there are some hidden contacts with contaminated water in the everyday life of the tourist and even some ways for bottled water to become tainted. To wit, take note of the following dos and don'ts:

**1.** Don't accept unsealed or uncapped bottled water. Open the seal yourself or have it opened in your presence. Carbonated water is safer than plain water.

**2.** Don't drink anything containing ice, ice cubes or ice water. This means no iced tea or coffee!

**3.** Don't drink reconstituted frozen, concentrated or powdered juices, reconstituted powdered milk or any other reconstituted drink unless it is mixed with bottled or boiled water in your presence.

**4.** Do drink directly from a bottle or can rather than from a questionable glass or cup. But if a can or bottle has been sitting on ice, wipe it clean and dry before drinking from it.

**5.** Do wash fruit with purified, boiled, or chemically sterilized water or, better yet, peel it before eating. Do stay away from raw vegetables, and don't eat salads prepared with raw fruits or vegetables.

**6.** Do choose only carbonated soft drinks. They're considered safer.

**7.** Do steer clear of street food vendors.

**8.** Do choose restaurants for their clean and sanitary looks.

**9.** Do drink only pasteurized milk. Use the helpful phrases on page 55. And don't trust milk or other dairy products in small villages or remote areas. Even in the larger cities, don't buy *any* dairy product from a street vendor. That includes ice cream, yogurt, and cheese.

# Spain

The water problems here are not as severe or as insidious as those in Mexico. Although drinking water in Spanish cities is chlorinated, it may contain bacteria that could bother you. That's because, though the water you drink back home has its own bacteria problems, your body *has* built up an immunity to the particular strains it contains. In Spain, you'll be making the acquaintance of their distant relatives, and it may take you a while to develop a harmonious relationship with them. If you're visiting Spain for just a short time, it may not pay to take this trouble when you can just as easily use bottled water for drinking and brushing your teeth. If you're planning a lengthy stay, however, drink the tap water and in time you and its new bacteria will develop a great friendship.

Milk and dairy products are pasteurized here, but if you do buy them in small towns, ask about pasteurization and refrigeration. You'll find some useful phrases on page 55. Although Spain's pasteurized milk is safe to drink, many people don't care for its flavor and recommend it only for cooking and baking. Or maybe coffee. Ice cream? There is some good news for weight watchers here. Milk is often used instead of cream in commercial ice creams in Spain.

A final word of caution about raw shellfish in both Mexico and Spain. Mexico has a parasite problem; be sure all shellfish is cooked well. In Spain, any shellfish caught in Mediterranian waters should be cooked well also; shellfish taken from northern waters may be eaten without this concern. If you're not sure of your dinner's origin, don't eat it unless you know it has been thoroughly cooked.

# Dining Out in Mexico and Spain

This section is divided into three parts. Part 1 includes a description of the hours for mealtimes, the available types of eating establishments, cover charges and tipping customs, plus some techniques of finding a restaurant and making reservations. Also, after finding a restaurant, there are questions included which you may need to ask, such as how to find a smoke-free spot. Part 2 gives some basic food lists arranged in breakfast, lunch, and dinner order. Part 3 contains a series of diet scenarios, each linked to specific health problems plus a scenario adaptable to the needs of travelers on special diets not covered in the more specific scenarios. Look them over now and check those items that will come in handy later.

## Part 1

In both Mexico and Spain, meals and coffee breaks take on a social aspect they don't have here in the United States. A luncheon for a Mexican or Spaniard can last from 2:00 P.M. to maybe 5:00 P.M. because during that time many conversations or business deals will take place. So too, a stop for *un café* (a cup of coffee) means sipping *several* cups of coffee, observing the diners around you and the passersby too (if you're at an outdoor cafe), discussing the day's events, and making future plans. All this proceeds at a very relaxed pace and may last for two or three hours.

## Mealtimes in Mexico

Travelers should be aware of the late lunch and dinner hours. If you arrive at a restaurant very early, you might get a standard-fare meal; the specialties of the day will not be ready until about 2:00 P.M.

Breakfast:  served between 8:00 and 10:30
Lunch:   served between 1:00 and 3:00
Dinner:  served from 8:00 until very late evening

# Types of Eating Establishments in Mexico

**Bar** — Bars are found in most of the better hotels and serve drinks and appetizers (*botanas*). Many of them feature musical entertainment.

**Café** — It's a coffee shop that can be found almost anywhere in Mexico. Some are very attractive, others more simple. They may serve sandwiches, cakes and pastries, herb and black teas, and soft drinks.

**Cafetería** — Vips, Dennys, Burger Boy, Sanborns—you'll see them everywhere. They are fast-food establishments with a Mexican twist in that they serve the traditional tacos, enchiladas, and tortas (those fabulous Mexican hard-roll sandwiches, which, unfortunately, usually contain the shredded raw lettuce we're supposed to stay away from in Mexico). The food is relatively inexpensive.

**Cantina** — These are for men only! These are bars but also good places to see a Mexican *campesino* or worker relaxing with a drink of *Pulque* (a gooey alcoholic beverage made from the agave cactus) or *tequila.*

**Fonda** — These are restaurants that serve *only* traditional Mexican food, which is usually very good.

**Hostería** — A restaurant that serves mostly traditional dishes and where regional specialties may be on the menu.

**Posada** — These are very similar to *fondas* and *hosterias.*

**Restaurante** — They are divided into these categories: *du lujo* (deluxe), *de primera* (first class), *de segunda* (second class), *de tercera* (third class). For the most part they serve specialty foods such as Italian, French, or Spanish food. Unfortunately, the *continental* or mixed cuisine restaurant is now hard to find.

**Restaurante de Carretera** — Pleasant establishments

usually located on the highways. They serve adequate meals and are usually clean.

*Taquerías* — Restaurants that specialize in all kinds of tacos. Some are clean, others are not, but the food is very good. A word of advice: avoid them unless a friend, who can vouch for the place, takes you.

# Tipping and Cover Charges in Mexico

Tips should be 15 percent of the bill. Sometimes they are included in the bill, but to be sure, read the menu very carefully, or ask the maitre d'. If a tip is included in the price of your meal, it will say *servicio incluído* on the menu. If you want to ask, say: *"¿Está incluído el servicio?"* You should also ask about a cover charge: *"¿Esta incluído el recargo?"*

# Mealtimes in Spain

Breakfast:   served between 7:30 and 10:30
Lunch:   served between 1:30 and 3:30
Dinner:   served between 9:30 and 11:00

For early-rising working people there are two breakfasts; the first, between 7:30 and 9:00, consists of coffee, hot chocolate, *churros* (fried crullers), rolls and jam, and fruit juice, usually fresh orange juice. Between 9:00 and 10:30 comes a hearty breakfast of bacon, sausages, eggs, coffee, chocolate, sweet rolls, toast and jam.

*Tapas* (hors d'oeuvres) are served between 1:00 and 2:00 with beer or wine. There are about 20 to 30 varieties of *tapas,* ranging from stewed quail to snails in hot sauce and tripe stew. If your stomach is delicate, avoid them; but if the thought doesn't put you off and your diet will allow it, by all means, visit a bar, café or tavern and enjoy a Spanish experience unknown in other European countries. The famous *tapa* bars in Madrid are in the neighborhood of *La Calle Echegaray* (Echegaray Street), named after a Spanish playwright and Nobel Prize winner.

Luncheon is the main meal in Spain, while dinner often resembles our lunch.

# Eating Establishments in Spain

**Bars** — Bars serve drinks, wine, beer, coffee, tapas (hors d'oeuvres), and sandwiches. They remain open until 1:00 or 2:00 A.M. Every town boasts several *bars;* there is one small town with 60 of them, each serving its own special *tapa.*

**Café** — A *café* is the same as a *bar* and open until 1:00 or 2:00 A.M.

**Cafeterías** — These are American-style eateries that serve breakfast, lunch, and supper and American or Spanish cuisine. They are very popular with Spanish young people. In Madrid you'll find them around the *Avenida José Antonio.* They are open until midnight or 1:00 A.M.

**Paradores** — *Paradores* are inns established by the Spanish Department of Tourism. Inquire about them while traveling in Spain by asking: *"¿Dónde está el parador más cercano?"* (Where is the nearest parador?) They are housed in ancient buildings, castles, abandoned convents, forgotten hospitals, and monasteries. Good food is available at reasonable prices. The atmosphere is delightful; the service excellent. They are exceptionally clean. Because the *paradores* are so popular, lodging is usually limited to two-night stays.

**Restaurantes** — Some serve breakfast but many do not open until lunchtime. They close between 11:00 P.M. and noon of the following day. As in Mexico they are divided into several categories, depending on the quality of their food and service. Most of them specialize in regional cooking, or French or Italian cooking.

**Tabernas** (taverns) — These are typical eating places, usually in low income neighborhoods. Some are very good and relatively inexpensive. They serve a variety of home-style meals.

# Tipping in Spain

Tips should be 15 percent of the bill. If the menu says *servicio incluído,* the tip is included in the price of the meal. If you want to ask about this, say: *"¿Está incluído el servicio?"*

# One Last Word

Eating plays a very important part in the life of every Spaniard, and the lunch meal, *la comida,* is especially important—so important that stores, businesses, and schools close down from 1:00 to 4:00 P.M. *La comida* is eaten in a relaxed atmosphere, quite the opposite of lunch hour in the States.

# Making Reservations in Mexican and Spanish Restaurants

Let the chef know you're coming and that you must observe a special diet. Ask your hotel manager or desk clerk to phone ahead for you. If you don't speak Spanish, and they don't speak English, simply point to the appropriate phrases.

Ask the desk clerk or hotel manager to read the following section before he or she phones for a reservation. To describe your needs, fill in the blanks with words and phrases selected from the "not permitted" list under your diet, the diet's scenario, the food lists, and the food preparation information in *Appendix 1.* Note that the symbol (M) next to an item indicates it is available only in Mexico. The symbol (S) indicates it is available only in Spain.

■ **Can you recommend a good, but not too expensive restaurant?**
¿Me podría usted recomendar un restaurante bueno, pero no muy caro?

■ **I have/she/he has a special problem and would like you to read the following:**

Tengo/tiene un problema médico y quisiera que usted leyera lo siguiente:

■ **I must ask a favor of you. I have/she/he has a medical problem and must observe a very special diet.**

Necesito pedirle un favor. Tengo/tiene un problema médico y debo/debe mantener una dieta rígida.

■ **Since I cannot speak Spanish, may I ask you to phone the restaurant for me and explain the problem?**

¿Como no sé hablar español, le sería posible hablar de mi parte al restaurante y explicarles mi/su problema?

■ **May I ask you to do a favor for me/for us? Please phone this restaurant and make a reservation for a party of _____ for me for lunch/dinner. For today/tomorrow. For Monday/Tuesday/Wednesday/Thursday/Friday/Saturday/Sunday. At _____ o'clock.**

¿Le puedo/podemos pedir un favor? Por favor hable usted a este restaurante y hágame/háganos una reservación para _____ personas para la comida/la cena. Para hoy/para mañana. El lunes /martes / miércoles /jueves /viernes /sábado/domingo a las _____ de la tarde/de la noche.

■ **I/she/he cannot eat anything containing _____.**

No puedo/puede tomar nada que contenga _____.

■ **If I eat/she/he eats _____ I/she/he can become seriously ill.**

Si tomo/toma algo que contenga _____ me/le podría causar una enfermedad muy grave.

- **Ask the maitre d' if he will be so kind as to arrange for simple substitutions in the dishes served to me.**
  Por favor pregúntele al maitre si le sería posible hacerles unas sustituciones muy sencillas a mis/ sus platillos.

- **For example, for lunch/dinner I would like _____ or _____.**
  Por ejemplo, para la comida (M), el almuerzo (S)/ la cena quiero/quiere _____ o _____.

- **It should be _____ (method of preparation – see Appendix 1).**
  Debe/deben ser _____.

- **It should not contain any _____.**
  No debe/deben contener nada de _____.

- **Please ask for the name of the person with whom you are speaking. Write it down (PRINT it) for me. Thank you very much.**
  Necesito saber el nombre de la persona con quien está usted hablando. Por favor escríbalo en LETRA DE MOLDE. Muchas gracias.

- **Please PRINT the name, address, and telephone number. Thank you.**
  Por favor escriba usted en LETRA DE MOLDE el nombre, la dirección y el teléfono. Gracias.

After the call has been made, you can ask:

- **Have you made the reservation?**
  ¿Pudo hacer las reservaciónes?

- **Did they understand my/her/his problem?**
  ¿Comprendiéron mi/su problema?

- **Are they willing to arrange for special dishes?**
  ¿Les será posible preparar los platillos requeridos?

You'll find these phrases helpful if you choose a restaurant on the spur of the moment.

■ **Are reservations necessary?**
¿Necesito hacer reservaciones?

■ **A table for _____, please. (See list of numbers on page 100.)**
Una mesa para _____ personas, por favor.

■ **Do you have a nonsmoking section?**
¿Tienen una sección de no fumar?

■ **Please, can you seat me/us as far away from smokers as possible?**
¿Por favor, le sería posible sentarme/sentarnos bastante lejos de los fumadores?

■ **I have/she/he has a serious allergy to smoke.**
Tengo/ella/él tiene una grave alergia al humo.

■ **Where is the ladies'/men's room?**
¿Dónde está el baño para damas/caballeros?

■ **Do you have _____?**
¿Tiene usted _____?

■ **I would like _____.**
Quisiera _____.

■ **Please give me _____.**
Por favor déme _____.

  ■ **glass of water (See pages 37–39 about water.)**
  un vaso de agua

  ■ **bottle of plain water sealed/unopened**
  una botella cerrada de agua

  ■ **bottle of carbonated water unopened**
  una botella cerrada de agua con gas

- **bottle of mineral water unopened**
  una botella cerrada de agua mineral
- **fork/knife/spoon/napkin/straws**
  un tenedor/un cuchillo/una cuchara/una servilleta/unos popotes (M), unas pajas (S)

# Part 2

The phrases and basic food lists in this section will be a big help in restaurants, supermarkets, and food stores. For a list of numbers, see page 100.

## Breakfast

Many hotels in Spain serve a continental breakfast, consisting of hot coffee and hot milk (which may be mixed together), buns or bread, butter, and jam. The larger hotels catering to an international clientele offer a wider selection for breakfast. In Mexico's larger hotels and in the major cities, you will find many familiar foods on the breakfast menu. Fresh fruit is always available as a breakfast dish in Mexico and Spain.

## Fruit Juices — Jugos de Frutas

Drink only freshly squeezed or canned juice in Mexico. Do not drink reconstituted frozen juice or any concentrate mixed with water unless it is mixed with bottled water in your presence. Be sure all bottled water is uncapped or unsealed in your presence.

- **Is this juice freshly squeezed?**
  ¿Este jugo, es recién hecho?

- **Has water been added to it?**
  ¿Se le agregó agua?

- **Is this juice prepared from concentrate/from frozen juice?**
¿Este jugo es concentrado o congelado?

- **I want only freshly squeezed/canned juice.**
Solo quiero jugo recién hecho/jugo enlatado.

- **Do you have _____?**
¿Tiene usted _____?

- **I would like _____.**
Quisiera _____.

- **Please give me _____.**
Por favor déme _____.

Select the juice you want from the following table, and ask for *jugo de* _____ (the juice of _____).

# Fruit Juices

*English—Spanish*
- apple—manzana
- apricot—chabacano (M), albaricoque (S)
- grape—uva
- grapefruit—toronja (M), pomelo (S)
- lemon—lima (M)*, limón (S)
- orange—naranja
- pear—pera
- pineapple—piña
- prune—ciruela seca
- tomato—tomate†

*Spanish-English*
- albaricoque (S)—apricot
- chabacano (M)—apricot
- ciruela seca—prune
- lima (M)—lemon*
- limón (S)—lemon
- manzana—apple
- naranja—orange
- pera—pear
- piña—pineapple
- pomelo (S)—grapefruit
- tomate—tomato†
- toronja (M)—grapefruit
- uva—grape

*The American yellow lemon or *lima* is hard to find in Mexico. Instead you will find *limón* or lime.

†Tomato or *tomate* in Mexico is a small green tomato used in many traditional sauces. Tomato as we know it in the United States is called *jitomate*.

# Fruit — Fruta

| English — Spanish | Spanish — English |
|---|---|
| ▪ apple—manzana | ▪ aceitunas—olives |
| ▪ applesauce—purée de manzana | ▪ albaricoques (S)—apricots |
| ▪ apricots—chabacanos (M), albaricoques (S) | ▪ aguacate (M)—avocado |
| ▪ avocado—aguacate (M) | ▪ cerezas (S)—cherries |
| ▪ banana—plátano | ▪ chabacanos (M)—apricots |
| ▪ cherries—cerezas (S) | ▪ ciruela—plum |
| ▪ coconut—coco | ▪ ciruelas secas—prunes |
| ▪ dates—dátiles | ▪ coco—coconut |
| ▪ figs—higos | ▪ dátiles—dates |
| ▪ grapefruit—toronja (M), pomelo (S) | ▪ durazno (M)—peach |
| ▪ grapes—uvas | ▪ fresas—strawberries* |
| ▪ grapes, seedless—uvas sin semillas | ▪ granada—pomegranate |
| ▪ guava—guayaba (M) | ▪ grosellas (S)—red currants |
| ▪ lemon—lima (M), limón (S) | ▪ guayaba (M)—guava |
| ▪ lime—limón (M), lima (S) | ▪ higos—figs |
| ▪ mango (M) | ▪ lima (M)—lemon |
| ▪ melon—melón | ▪ lima (S)—lime |
| ▪ olives—aceitunas | ▪ limón (M)—lime |
| ▪ orange—naranja | ▪ limón (S)—lemon |
| ▪ peach—durazno (M), melocotón (S) | ▪ mandarina—tangerine |
| ▪ pear—pera | ▪ mango (M) |
| ▪ pineapple—piña (M) | ▪ manzana—apple |
| ▪ plum—ciruela | ▪ melocotón (S)—peach |
| ▪ pomegranate—granada | ▪ melón—melon |
| ▪ prunes—ciruelas secas | ▪ membrillo—quince |
| ▪ raisins—pasas | ▪ naranja—orange |
| ▪ red currants—grosellas (S) | ▪ pasas—raisins |
| ▪ quince—membrillo | ▪ pera—pear |
| ▪ strawberries—fresas* | ▪ piña (M)—pineapple |
| ▪ tangerine—mandarina | ▪ plátano—banana |
| ▪ watermelon—sandía | ▪ pomelo (S)—grapefruit |
| | ▪ purée de manzana— applesauce |
| | ▪ sandía—watermelon |
| | ▪ toronja (M)—grapefruit |
| | ▪ uvas—grapes |
| | ▪ uvas sin semillas— seedless grapes |

*Never eat strawberries in Mexico. As a rule of thumb, don't eat anything you cannot peel. But strawberries in Spain are another matter. They are excellent in early summer. *Fresas* are small and wild; *fresones* are the large, cultivated berries.

If you want new and different taste sensations, try these tropical fruits in Mexico and Spain:

*chirimoya*—white with black seeds and very tasty

*nísperos*—tart, aromatic flavor, with large seeds in the center

The following fruits are available only in Mexico, and most of them are found only in markets.

*capulín*—small sour cherries

*chico zapote*—small, brownish skin with orange-colored pulp; pleasant, sweet flavor

*granada china*—a strange fruit for the more adventurous. The exterior is a hard, orange-colored shell, which you cut away as if you were peeling a soft-boiled egg. Inside is a delicious, gooey, seedy pulp. The seeds are edible but many spit them out.

*guayaba*—like a guava; seedy, with creamy texture

*higos*—fresh figs, not the dried or canned figs that can also be found in both Mexico and Spain. They are either green or black. Both varieties are delicious and totally different from canned or dried figs. You won't find these in restaurants although canned figs are often served as a dessert in restaurants.

*jicama*—a crisp root similar to a water chestnut; often served with lemon juice as an appetizer

*mamey*—very sweet and creamy with an aromatic flavor; excellent blended with milk

*mango*—contains a large pit; the yellow pulp is very aromatic and sweet. In Mexican restaurants canned mangos are often made into desserts such as mango cream or mango pie.

*papaya*—a mild fruit, easily digestible; a sweet, aromatic flavor; often served for breakfast

*pitahaya*—very sweet with crunchy small seeds throughout fruit

*tamarindo*—very tart; exterior shell must be peeled

*tejocote*—a type of crab apple

*tuna (prickly pear)*—sweet, juicy, refreshingly crisp; very seedy

*zapote negro*—bright green on the outside; inside it is brownish black; not very attractive but quite tasty—often mixed with orange juice. If ripe, it is soft to the touch.

**Attention:** If you are on a bland diet, you can try some of these fruits but minus the skin and seeds. Of the exotic fruits, the following are suggested for bland diets by Mexico's Instituto Nacional de la Nutricion: *chirimoya, chico zapote, mamey, papaya* and *zapote.*

Now that you've had your fruit juice and/or fruit, you're ready for the next course. Have a hearty breakfast. It will keep you sightseeing for hours and stave off the hunger that may trap you into stuffing yourself at dinner. If your hotel offers only continental breakfasts and you want something more substantial, speak with the hotel manager or the maitre d' the day or evening before your first morning meal. Try these phrases:

■ **May I ask a special favor of you?**
   ¿Le puedo pedir un favor?

■ **Would it be possible to have _____ for breakfast?**
   ¿Le sería posible traerme _____ para el desayuno?

Select something from the following lists of breakfast foods, but keep it simple. If necessary, show your WALLET CARD; it will lend authority to your request. If your food must be prepared in a special way, point to the appropriate phrases (*Appendix 1*). Better still, put it all down on paper before you approach the maitre d'. PRINT it! Of course, you'll feel a little silly and embarrassed the very first time you flash your WALLET CARD and make a special request. Who wouldn't? But keep in mind that the hotel staff is anxious to make your stay a comfortable one. The important thing is to be polite and friendly in making your request. After you've tried it once, you'll become an old hand at it. Okay, let's get back to breakfast.

# Cereals – Cereales

You can get some cold cereals in restaurants in Mexico, but you will have a hard time finding them in Spanish restaurants. No translation is needed for the following

three cold cereals. Ask for:
All Bran
Cornflakes
Rice Krispies

## Hot Cereals—Cereales Calientes

■ **Please cook it in unsalted water.**

Por favor, hiérvalo en agua sin sal.

Hot cereals are rarely eaten for breakfast in Spain. If you are ordering cereal in Mexico, you'll want to be sure the water has been boiled for at least ten minutes.

■ **Please boil the water for at least ten minutes.**

Por favor, hierva el agua por lo menos diez minutos.

■ **Don't put any _____ in it.**

No le ponga _____.

■ **Please put some _____ in it.**

Por favor póngale _____.

■ **Do you have _____?**

¿Tiene usted _____?

■ **I would like _____.**

Quisiera _____.

■ **Please give me _____.**

Por favor déme _____.

The following cereals are sometimes available in restaurants:
• barley—cebada perla
• oatmeal—avena
• bran—salvado
• brown rice—arroz integral
• buckwheat—trigo negro
• cornmeal—fécula de maíz
• millet—mijo

- rye—centeno
- soy—soya (M), soja (S)
- wheat germ—germen de trigo
- white rice—arroz blanco
- whole wheat—trigo integral

If your digestive problem requires a highly refined cereal, ask:

■ **Do you have refined cereals suitable for babies?**
¿Tienen ustedes cereales refinados tipo "Pablum" para bebé?

## Bread, Rolls, Crackers, and Pancakes—Pan, Panecillos, Galletas, y Hot Cakes

- corn—de maíz
- rye—de centeno
- soy—de soya (M), de soja (S)
- white—blanco
- whole wheat—integral

■ **Please toast the bread.**
Por favor, quiero el pan tostado.

■ **Please warm the _____.**
Por favor, caliente el/la/los/las _____.
- bread—pan
- crackers—galletas [If you are on a low-sodium or bland diet, you might enjoy crackers called *María galletas* (M).]
- muffins—panecillos
- pancakes—in Mexico ask for *hot cakes.*
- rolls—bolillo (M), panecillo (S)
- tortillas—tortillas (M) (Remember, in Mexico a tortilla is a thin flat pancake, usually made from cornmeal. A tortilla in Spain is an omelet. If you ask for *una tortilla de huevo sencilla* in Mexico, you will get a plain omelet.)

# Eggs — Huevos

- fried — estrellados (M), fritos (S)
- hard-boiled — duros
- poached — escalfados, poché
- scrambled — revueltos
- soft-boiled — tibios

# Dairy Products — Productos Lácteos

■ **Is it pasteurized?**
¿Es pasteurizado/a?

■ **Has it been refrigerated?**
¿Se mantuvo en refrigeración?

- butter — mantequilla
- unsalted butter — mantequilla sin sal
- margarine — margarina
- made from vegetable oil — hecha de aceite vegetal de

  - corn — maíz
  - peanut — cacahuate (M), cacahuete (S)
  - safflower — cártamo
  - soy — soya (M), soja (S)
  - sunflower — girasol (S)

## *Cheese — Queso and Yogurt — Yogurt*

■ **Is it made with whole milk?**
¿Fue hecho con leche entera?

■ **Is it made with skim milk?**
¿Fue hecho con leche descremada?

■ **Is it made with part skim milk?**
¿Fue hecho con leche parcialmente descremada?

■ **Has salt/sugar/sweetening been added?**
¿Se le agregó sal/azúcar/endulzante?

■ **Has cream been added?**
¿Se le agregó crema (M)/nata (S)?

■ **Is it creamed?**
¿Es queso crema?

■ **What percentage of fat does it contain?**
¿Cuál es el porcentage de grasa?

■ **Please write it down. Thank you.**
Por favor, escríbalo. Gracias.

■ **Do you have a cheese/yogurt that is _____?**
¿Tiene usted algún queso/yogurt _____?
  • low-calorie—bajo en calorías
  • low-fat—bajo en grasa
  • low-salt—bajo en sal

In Mexico, low-fat cottage cheese contains 4 percent fat;
a semi-low-fat processed cottage cheese has 17 percent fat.

### Cream—Crema (M), Nata (S)
  • nondairy creamer—artificial
  • sour—agria
  • sweet—dulce

### Milk—Leche
  • buttermilk—jocoque (M)
  • condensed milk—leche condensada
  • evaporated milk—leche evaporada
  • evaporated skim milk—leche evaporada descremada
  • evaporated whole milk—leche evaporada entera
  • fresh skim—descremada fresca
  • fresh whole—entera fresca
  • homogenized—homogenizada

- not homogenized—sin homogenizar
- kefir—leche búlgara
- pasteurized—pasteurizada
- powdered skim—descremada en polvo
- powdered whole—entera en polvo
- boiled for at least ten minutes—hervida por lo menos diez minutos

If you ask for powdered milk in Mexico, remember the precautions about the water used to reconstitute the milk.

# Spreads

- honey—miel de abeja (rarely found in Spanish restaurants)
- jam—mermelada
- jelly—jalea
- marmalade—mermelada de naranja
- peanut butter—mantequilla de cacahuate (M), de cacahuete (S)
  - chunky—con trocitos
  - freshly ground—recién hecha
  - plain/smooth—cremosa/sin trocitos
  - salt-free—sin sal
  - sugar-free (no sweetening)—sin endulzante
  - unhydrogenated—sin hidrogenar
  - without additives—sin aditivos

# Beverages—Bebidas

You might want something to wash down that substantial breakfast.
- chocolate (cocoa)—chocolate caliente (Mexican and Spanish cocoa contains vanilla and cinnamon.)
- coffee—café
- decaffeinated coffee—café descafeinado
- a glass of milk—un vaso de leche
- a glass of skim milk—un vaso de leche descremada
- chocolate milk—una leche fría con chocolate

- malted milk—una leche malteada de _____:
  - vanilla—vainilla
  - chocolate—chocolate
  - strawberry—fresa (Remember, no fresh strawberries in Mexico! Strawberry jam, preserves, or jelly—as long as the berries have been cooked—are okay.)
- tea—té
- herb tea—té de _____ (M), infusión de _____ (S)
  - camomile—manzanilla
  - cinnamon—canela
  - linden—tila
  - spearmint—yerba buena

For an additional listing of beverages, see pages 70–72.

## Lunch and Dinner

Worried about preparation? Consult *Appendix 1: Spanish Food Preparation.*

Here are a few tips about meat in Mexico. You'll find the flavor of Mexican beef different from our homemade variety. Veal is popular. Lamb? Rarely found on menus. In Spain, the beef isn't very tasty, and you'll find veal closer in flavor to American beef. Game is abundant in Spain from late autumn through Christmas and many excellent dishes are prepared with partridges and other wild birds.

If you are curious about the meat in a dish on a menu, ask:

■ **What kind of meat is this?**
¿Qué tipo de carne es ésta?

■ **Please show me on this list.**
Por favor enséñeme en esta lista.

■ **I would like** _____.
Quiero _____.

- beef—res (M), vaca (S)
- chicken—pollo
- lamb—carnero (M), cordero (S)
- lean meat—carne magra (Remember, if you want lean cuts, be sure to add the word *magra*.)
- pork—cerdo (M), puerco (S)
- turkey—pavo
- veal—ternera

Here are some cuts of meat, listed by category—beef, lamb, pork, poultry, veal, and variety meats.

# Cuts of Meat

*English—Spanish*
**Beef—*Res (M), Vaca (S)***

- cutlet—milanesa de res (M), escalope de vaca (S)
- eye of the round roast—cuete de res (M), redondo de vaca (S)
- ground beef—carne molida de res (M), carne picada de vaca (S)
- liver—hígado (Liver is lean but *high* in cholesterol.)
- oxtail—rabo de buey, cola de buey
- roast beef—rosbif (M)
- short ribs—costillas cortas (M), agujas (M)
- steak—bistec de res (M), bistec de vaca (S)
  - Delmonico—costilla de rosbif (M)

*Spanish—English*
***Res (M), Vaca (S)—*Beef**

- agujas (M)—short ribs
- bistec de filete (M)—tenderloin steak
- bistec de res—beef steak (M)
- bistec de vaca—beef steak (S)
- callos—tripe
- carne molida de res (M)—ground beef
- carne picada de vaca (S)—ground beef
- cola de buey—oxtail
- contra filete de vaca (S)—T-bone steak
- costilla de rosbif (M)—Delmonico steak
- costillas cortas (M)—short ribs
- cuete de res (M)—eye of the round roast

*(continued on next page)*

# Cuts of Meat  (continued)

*English—Spanish*
**Beef—*Res (M), Vaca (S)*
(continued)**

- flank steak—falda de res (M), falda de vaca (S)
- small steak similar to fillet—diezmillo (M)
- T-bone—tibón, T-bone (M), contra filete de vaca (S)
- tenderloin steak—bistec de filete (M), solomillo de vaca (S)
- tenderloin chunks—puntas de filete (M), solomillo de vaca en trozos (S)
- tenderloin roast—filete de res (M), solomillo de vaca (S)
- tripe—pancita (M), callos (S)

*Spanish—English*
***Res (M), Vaca (S)*—Beef**

- diezmillo (M)—small steak similar to fillet
- escalope de vaca (S)—cutlet
- falda de res (M)—flank steak
- falda de vaca (S)—flank steak
- filete de res (M)—tenderloin roast
- hígado—liver
- milanesa de res (M)—beef cutlet
- pancita (M)—tripe
- puntas de filete (M)—tenderloin chunks
- rabo de buey—oxtail
- redondo de vaca (S)—eye of the round roast
- rosbif (M)—roast beef
- solomillo de vaca (S)—beef tenderloin, tenderloin roast
- solomillo de vaca en trozos (S)—tenderloin chunks
- tibón—T-bone steak (M)

**Lamb—*Carnero (M), Cordero (S)***

- chop—chuleta de carnero (M), chuleta de cordero (S)
- leg—pierna de carnero (M), pierna de cordero (S)

***Carnero (M), Cordero (S)*—Lamb**

- chuleta de carnero (M)—chop
- chuleta de cordero (S)—chop
- espaldilla de carnero (M)—shoulder roast

## English—Spanish

- shank—jarrete de carnero (M), jarrete de cordero (S)
- shoulder roast—espaldilla de carnero (M), paletilla de cordero (S)

## Spanish—English

- jarrete de carnero (M)— shank
- jarrete de cordero (S)— shank
- paletilla de cordero (S)— shoulder roast
- pierna de carnero (M)— leg
- pierna de cordero (S)— leg

**Pork—Cerdo (M), Puerco (S)**

- chop—chuleta de cerdo (M), chuleta de puerco (S)
- cutlet—milanesa de cerdo (M), escalope de puerco (S)
- ground pork—carne molida de cerdo (M), carne picada de puerco (S)
- ham—jamón
  - cured ham—jamón serrano (excellent— lean; a "must" in Spain)
  - fresh ham—tierna de puerco
  - leg—pierna de jamón
  - shank—jarrete de jamón
  - smoked ham (center slices)—jamón ahumado (rebanadas del centro)
- loin roast—lomo de cerdo (M), lomo de puerco (S)
- ribs—costillas de cerdo (M), costillas de puerco (S)

**Cerdo (M), Puerco (S)—Pork**

- bien recortado—well- trimmed
- carne molida de cerdo (M)—ground meat
- carne picada de puerco (S)—ground meat
- chuleta ahumada— smoked chop
- chuleta de cerdo (M)— chop
- chuleta de puerco (S)— chop
- cochinillo—suckling pig
- costillas de cerdo (M)— ribs
- costillas de puerco (S)— ribs
- filete de cerdo (M)— tenderloin
- jamón ahumado (rebanadas del centro)— smoked ham (center slices)
- jamón serrano—cured ham
- jarrete de jamón—ham shank

*(continued on next page)*

# Cuts of Meat  (continued)

*English—Spanish*
**Pork—*Cerdo (M)*,
*Puerco (S)*
*(continued)***
- smoked chop—chuleta ahumada
- suckling pig—lechón, cochinillo
- tenderloin—filete de cerdo (M), solomillo de puerco (S)
- tenderloin chunks of pork—puntas de filete de cerdo (M), solomillo de puerco en trozos (S)
- well-trimmed—bien recortado

*Spanish—English*
***Cerdo (M), Puerco (S)*
—Pork**
- escalope de puerco—cutlet (S)
- filete de cerdo (M)—tenderloin
- jamón—ham
- lechón—suckling pig
- lomo de cerdo (M)—loin roast
- lomo de puerco (S)—loin roast
- milanesa de cerdo (M)—cutlet
- pierna de jamón—ham leg
- puntas de filete de cerdo (M)—tenderloin chunks
- solomillo de puerco (S)—tenderloin
- solomillo de puerco en trozos (S)—tenderloin chunks
- tierna de puerco—fresh ham

**Poultry—*Aves***
- capon—capón (S)
- chicken—pollo
  - breast—pechuga
  - leg—pierna
  - roast chicken—pollo asado
  - thigh—muslo
  - wing—ala
- duck/duckling—pato
- goose—ganso (S)
- partridge—perdiz
- pheasant—faisán (S)

***Aves*—Poultry**
- capón—capon
- codorniz (S)—quail
- faisán—pheasant
- ganso (S)—goose
- pato—duck/duckling
- pavo—turkey
  - ala—wing
  - muslo—thigh
  - pavo asado—roast turkey
  - pechuga—breast
  - pierna—leg

## English—Spanish
- pigeon—pichón
- quail—codorniz (S)
- turkey—pavo
  - breast—pechuga
  - leg—pierna
  - roast turkey—pavo asado
  - thigh—muslo
  - wing—ala

## Spanish—English
- perdiz—partridge
- pichón—pigeon
- pollo—chicken
  - ala—wing
  - muslo—thigh
  - pechuga—breast
  - pierna—leg
  - pollo asado—roast chicken

## Veal—*Ternera*
- chop—chuleta de ternera
- cutlet—milanesa de ternera (M), escalope de ternera (S)
- eye of the round roast— cuete de ternera (M), redondo de ternera (S)
- ground veal—carne molida de ternera (M), carne picada de ternera (S)
- kidney chops—chuletas de ternera con riñón
- shank—jarrete de ternera
- steak—bistec de ternera
  - flank steak—falda de ternera
  - T-bone—tibón de ternera (M), contra filete de ternera (S)
- tenderloin roast—filete de ternera (M), solomillo de ternera (S)

## *Ternera*—Veal
- bistec de ternera—steak
- carne molida de ternera (M)—ground meat
- carne picada de ternera (S)—ground meat
- chuletas de ternera con riñón—kidney chops
- chuleta de ternera— chop
- contra filete de ternera (S)—T-bone steak
- cuete de ternera (M)— eye of the round roast
- escalope de ternera (S)— cutlet
- falda de ternera—flank steak
- filete de ternera (M)— tenderloin
- jarrete de ternera—shank
- milanesa de ternera (M)— cutlet
- redondo de ternera (S)— eye of the round roast
- solomillo de ternera (S)— tenderloin roast

## Other Meats and Variety Meats
- bacon—tocino
- blood sausage— mondongo (M), morcillas (S)

- cabrito—goat/kid
- carne picada—minced meat

*(continued on next page)*

# Cuts of Meat (continued)

*English—Spanish*

**Other Meats and Variety Meats**

- brains—sesos
- chicken livers—higaditos de pollo
- goat/kid—cabrito
- hare/wild rabbit—liebre
- kidneys—riñones
- minced meat—carne picada
- oxtail—rabo de buey, cola de buey
- pig's feet—manitas de cerdo (M), patitas de puerco (S)
- rabbit—conejo
- sausages—salchichas
- sweetbreads—mollejas de ternera (M), lechecillas (S)
- tongue—lengua
- venison—venado

*Spanish—English*

- cola de buey—oxtail
- conejo—rabbit
- higaditos de pollo— chicken livers
- lechecillas (S)— sweetbreads
- lengua—tongue
- liebre—hare/wild rabbit
- manitas de cerdo (M)— pig's feet
- mollejas de ternera (M)— sweetbreads
- mondongo (M)—blood sausage
- morcillas (S)—blood sausage
- patitas de puerco (S)— pig's feet
- rabo de buey—oxtail
- riñones—kidneys
- salchichas—sausages
- sesos—brains
- tocino—bacon
- venado—venison

# Fish—Pescado and Shellfish—Mariscos

- **What kind of fish is this?**
  ¿Qué tipo de pescado es este?

- **Please show me on this list.**
  Por favor enséñeme en esta lista.

- **Is it fresh?**
  ¿Es fresco?

- **Has it been frozen and thawed?**
  ¿Se ha congelado y descongelado?

- **Do you have _____?**
  ¿Tiene usted _____?

- **I would like _____.**
  Quisiera _____.

- **Please give me _____.**
  Por favor, déme _____.

# Fresh and Saltwater Fish

*English—Spanish*
- anchovies—anchoas (salty), boquerones (fresh)
- bass, striped—mero (M), lubina (S)
- bonito—bonito (very tasty)
- clams—almejas
- cod—bacalao
- conger eel—congrio (S) (very tasty)
  - small river eel—angula (M), anguila (S)
- crab—cangrejo
- crawfish—langostinos
- crayfish—cigalas
- flounder—lenguado
- goose barnacles—percebes (expensive in Spain and found only in restaurants)
- haddock—robalo
- hake—merluza (excellent fish in Spain; try it cooked any Basque style)

*Spanish—English*
- abadejo (S)—pollock
- almejas—clams
- anchoas—anchovies (salty)
- anguila (S)—eel
- angula (M)—eel
- arenque—herring
- atún—tuna
- bacalao—cod
- bagre—sawfish
- besugo (S)—sea bream
- bonito—bonito
- boquerones—anchovies (fresh)
- calamares—squid
- callos de hacha (M)—scallops
- camarón—shrimp
- camarones (M)—prawns
- cangrejo—crab
- chipirones (S)—baby squid
- cigalas—crayfish
- congrio (S)—conger eel
- gambas (S)—prawns

*(continued on next page)*

## Fresh and Saltwater Fish
(continued)

*English—Spanish*
- herring—arenque
- lamprey—lamprea (S)
- lobster—langosta
- mackerel—macarela (M), jureles (S)
- monkfish—rape (S)
- mullet, gray—lisa
- mullet, red—salmonete
- mussels—mejillones
- octopus—pulpo
- oysters—ostiones (M), ostras (S)
- pollock—abadejo (S)
- porgy—pargo
- prawns—camarones (M), gambas (S)
- salmon—salmón (rare in Mexico, very expensive in Spain, but found in excellent restaurants)
  - smoked salmon— salmón ahumado
- sardines—sardinas (a must in Spain, fried or broiled)
- sawfish—bagre, pez sierra
- scallops—callos de hacha (M), vieira (S)
- sea bream— huachinango (M), besugo (S) (a Mediterranean type of red snapper)
- shrimp—camarón
- sole—lenguado
- squid—calamares
  - baby squid— chipirones (S)

*Spanish—English*
- huachinango—sea bream
- jureles (S)—mackerel
- lamprea (S)—lamprey
- langosta—lobster
- langostinos—crawfish
- lenguado—flounder, sole
- lisa—gray mullet
- lubina (S)—striped bass
- macarela (M)—mackerel
- mejillones—mussels
- merluza—hake
- mero (M)—striped bass
- ostiones (M)—oysters
- ostras (S)—oysters
- pargo—porgy
- percebes—goose barnacles
- pescadilla—whiting
- pez espada—swordfish
- pez sierra—sawfish
- pulpo—octopus
- rape (S)—monkfish
- robalo—haddock
- rodaballo—turbot
- salmón—salmon
- salmón ahumado— smoked salmon
- salmonete—red mullet
- tortuga (M)—turtle
- trucha de río—brook trout
- vieira (S)—scallops

*English—Spanish*
- swordfish—pez espada
- trout, brook—trucha de río
- tuna—atún
- turbot—rodaballo
- turtle, green—tortuga (M)
- whiting—pescadilla

*Spanish—English*

# Vegetables—Verduras

- **Do you have _____?**
  ¿Tiene usted _____?

- **I would like _____.**
  Quisiera _____.

- **Please give me _____.**
  Por favor déme _____.

# Vegetables

*English—Spanish*
- artichokes—alcachofas
- asparagus—espárragos
- brussels sprouts—coles de bruselas
- cabbage—col (M), repollo (S)
  - red cabbage—col morada (M), lombarda (S)
- capers—alcaparras (a bud used as a seasoning)
- carrots—zanahorias
- cauliflower—coliflor
- celery—apio
- chick-peas—garbanzos
- chicory—escarola

*Spanish—English*
- acelgas—Swiss chard
- ajo—garlic
- alcachofas—artichokes
- alcaparras—capers
- apio—celery
- arróz—rice
- batatas (S)—yams, sweet potatoes
- berenjena—eggplant
- calabacines (S)—zucchini
- calabacitas (M)—zucchini
- camotes (M)—yams, sweet potatoes
- cebollas—onion
- cebolletas—chives
- chícharos (M)—peas
- chiles (M)—hot peppers

*(continued on next page)*

67

# Vegetables *(continued)*

| English—Spanish | Spanish—English |
|---|---|
| chili—chile (M), pimientos picantes (S) | chirivia—parsnip |
| chives—cebolletas | col (M)—cabbage |
| corn—maiz (S) | coles de bruselas— brussels sprouts |
| corn on the cob—elote (M) | coliflor—cauliflower |
| cucumber—pepino | col morada (M)—red cabbage |
| eggplant—berenjena | ejotes (M)—green beans |
| garlic—ajo | elote (M)—corn on the cob |
| gherkins—encurtidos (M), pepinillos dulces (S) | encurtidos (M)—pickles, gherkins |
| green beans—ejotes (M), judías verdes (S) | escarola—chicory |
| leeks—poros (M), puerros (S) | espárragos—asparagus |
| lentils—lentejas | espinacas—spinach |
| lettuce—lechuga | garbanzos—chick-peas |
| mushrooms—hongos (M), setas (S) | guisantes (S)—peas |
| onions—cebollas | hongos (M)—mushrooms |
| parsley—perejil | jitomate—tomato* |
| parsnip—chirivía | judías verdes (S)—green beans |
| peas—chícharos (M), guisantes (S) | lechuga—lettuce |
| peppers, green or red— pimientos verdes o rojos | lentejas—lentils |
| pickles, gherkins— encurtidos (M) | lombarda (S)—red cabbage |
| potatoes—papas (M), patatas (S) | maíz—corn (S) |
| radishes—rábanos | nabo—turnip |
| rice—arróz | papas (M)—potatoes |
| spinach—espinacas | patatas (S)—potatoes |
| sweet peppers—pimientos | pepinillos dulces (S)— gherkins |
| sweet potatoes— camotes (M), batatas (S) (in Spain, used as a dessert and is hard to find in restaurants) | pepino—cucumber |
| | perejil—parsley |
| | pimientos—sweet peppers |
| | pimientos picantes (S)— hot peppers |

*Tomato or *tomate* in Mexico is a small green tomato used in many traditional sauces. Tomato as we know it in the United States is called *jitomate.*

| English—Spanish | Spanish—English |
|---|---|
| ■ Swiss chard—acelgas | ■ pimientos verdes o rojos —green or red peppers |
| ■ tomato—tomate* | ■ poros (M)—leeks |
| ■ truffles—trufas | ■ puerros (S)—leeks |
| ■ turnip—nabo | ■ rábanos—radishes |
| ■ yams—camotes (M), batatas (S) | ■ repollo (S)—cabbage |
| ■ zucchini—calabacitas (M), calabacines (S) | ■ setas (S)—mushrooms |
| | ■ tomate—tomato* |
| | ■ trufas—truffles |
| | ■ zanahorias—carrots |

## Pasta—Pasta

■ **Please cook it in unsalted water.**

Por favor cocínela en agua sin sal.

■ **Was this cooked in salted water?**

¿Se hirvió esto en agua salada?

■ **Please ask the chef to check the label on the container. Does it contain any _____?**

Por favor pídale al chef que lea la etiqueta del paquete. ¿Contiene _____?

- egg—huevo
- salt—sal
- sugar—azúcar
- sweetening—endulzante

### Pasta Products

- canelones (M)—like lasagna, but rolled and filled; rare in Spain
- lasagna—lasagna (M) (rare in Spain)
- macaroni—macarrones
- noodles—tallarines
- pastina—pastina
- spaghetti—espagueti (M), fideos (S)

*Tomato or *tomate* in Mexico is a small green tomato used in many traditional sauces. Tomato as we know it in the United States is called *jitomate*.

- spinach noodles—tallarines verdes
- vermicelli—vermicelli, fideos
- white flour—harina
- whole wheat flour—harina integral

## Nonalcoholic Beverages — Bebidas Analcohólicas

■ **Do you have _____?**
¿Tiene usted _____?

■ **I would like _____.**
Quisiera _____.

■ **Please give me _____.**
Por favor déme _____.

If you would like a glass of fruit juice, you can ask for *jugo de fruta* (juice of the fruit). In Spain, you may use the word *jugo* or *zumo;* in Mexico, only *jugo.*
- apple—manzana
- grape—uva
- grapefruit—toronja (M), pomelo (S)
- orange—naranja
- papaya—papaya
- pear—pera
- pineapple—piña

For a larger selection of fruit juices, see page 49.
Cola drinks can be ordered by their American names. Soft, carbonated drinks are *refrescos. Refrescos,* bottled fruit drinks, come in different flavors and can be loaded with sugar as well as additives and preservatives. Some popular flavors are:
- apple—manzana
- lemon—limón
- orange—naranja

Other nonalcoholic beverages you can order are:

- chocolate or cocoa (hot)—chocolate caliente
- coffee—café
  - café Americano (M)—American-style coffee
  - café Cappuchino—espresso with steamed milk plus a dash of cinnamon
  - café con leche—coffee with milk
  - café de olla (M)—prepared in a ceramic crock; boiled coffee with added cloves, cinnamon, natural brown sugar, and sometimes a dash of brandy or other liquor
  - café Espresso
  - café Irlandés—Irish coffee
- milk—leche; skim milk—leche descremada
- milk shake—leche malteada
- mineral water—agua mineral
- tea—té
  - té con leche—tea with milk
  - té con limón—tea with lemon
  - té negro—regular tea
- herb tea—té de _____ (M), infusión de _____ (S)
  - camomile—manzanilla
  - cinnamon—canela
  - linden—tila
  - spearmint—yerba buena
- tonic water—agua quina (M), tónica (S)

# Wines — Vinos

- red wine—vino tinto
- rosé—vino rosado
- white wine—vino blanco

■ **I want a light/dry/sweet/bubbly wine.**
Quiero un vino ligero/seco/dulce/espumoso.

■ **I want a glass of the white/red house wine.**
Quiero una copa del vino blanco/tinto de la casa.

## Alcoholic Drinks – Bebidas Alcohólicas

- anis-flavored liqueur—anís
- beer—cerveza
  - light—clara
  - dark—oscura (S)
- bourbon—borbón
- cognac—cognac
- gin—ginebra
- gin and tonic—ginebra con tónica
- gin fizz—ginebra con limón
- rum—ron
- rum Coke—Cuba libre
- Scotch—escocés
- sherry—jerez
- vermouth—vermut
- vodka—vodka
- whiskey—wisky
- whiskey and soda—wisky con soda

# Part 3

## For All Diets...

The Mexican and Spanish terms for most foods are identical. Where they differ, the symbols (M) and (S) next to the words will distinguish the pair. Where only one word and one symbol appear, the item is available only in one country, either Mexico or Spain.

A word of caution: Knorr Swiss seasoning is used in many Mexican dishes, including most soups. Among other ingredients, this seasoning contains monosodium glutamate (MSG) and beef or chicken fat. If you must avoid MSG, salt, or highly seasoned foods, be sure to include Knorr Swiss in your list of "not permitted" items. The words are similar in Spanish: *Knorr Suiza.*

Another commonly used flavoring in Mexico is *Rosa Blanca.* Sugar and salt are two of its ingredients and so if these are no-nos for you, add *Rosa Blanca* to your "not permitted" list.

# The Low-Sodium (Low-Salt) Diet

The following list of "not permitted" items may vary from the list your physician has instructed you to avoid. To make the list easier for others to read, cross out the items that do not apply to you and write in, PRINTING LEGIBLY, any other things you must avoid. Select them from the food lists on pages 48–72.

To make sure your food and drinks are prepared properly, consult *Appendix 1: Spanish Food Preparation.* Use it together with other appropriate pages when ordering meals.

Keep in mind these hidden sodium sources: baked goods may be made with baking powder (sodium bicarbonate) rather than yeast. Ask:

■ **Is this made with yeast?**

¿Fue hecho con levadura?

■ **Is this made with baking powder/baking soda?**

¿Fue hecho con polvo de hornear/bicarbonato de sodio?

Since *levadura* means leavening as well as yeast, your listener may misunderstand your question. Be sure to ask both of the preceding questions.

Beware also that antacids, like Alka Seltzer, and other indigestion aids may contain sodium bicarbonate or other sodium compounds. Before you go to Mexico or Spain, ask your physician to suggest a low-sodium antacid to take along. If you must buy an antacid, here's the Spanish for sodium bicarbonate or bicarbonate of soda: *bicarbonato de soda.* The names of other sodium compounds will have the word *sodio* in them. Look for it on labels. Also, if you must keep to a diet of less than 800 milligrams of sodium a day, don't use softened water. Ask:

■ **Does this water/the water in the hotel pass through a filter that softens it/removes the hard minerals?**
¿El agua del hotel, pasa por un filtro para suavizarla y quitarle los minerales?

Also check the labels on bottled water for sodium content. If the label does not contain a chemical analysis, use the table on page 27 as a guideline.

So far all you've read is *avoid, not permitted, beware,* and you're wondering what you can eat and drink in Mexico and Spain and still stick to your diet. Unfortunately, your diet scenario will sound pretty negative too, but don't let that frighten you. Take a look at the extensive food lists in *Part 2* of this section, pages 48–72. If you can't order from the menu the waiter gives you, ask for items on these food lists. Modify your selections with help from *Appendix 1: Spanish Food Preparation* and the diet scenario that follows for a satisfying meal, one custom-made to your specifications.

If you are staying at a Mexican hotel and plan to have most of your meals there, you can ask the maitre d' to stock Lonalac, a low-sodium powdered milk, for you. Just be sure boiled or bottled water is used to reconstitute the milk. You can get Lonalac at most pharmacies, and some large supermarkets may have it. A low-sodium biscuit is also available in Mexico. These biscuits *(galletas)* are called *Marías.*

---

# Foods Not Permitted – Alimentos Prohibidos

- anchovies—anchoas
- anything baked with baking powder or with baking soda—todo asado con bicarbonato de soda o polvo de hornear
- bacon fat—manteca de tocino
- baking soda—bicarbonato de soda

- celery salt—sal de ápio
- cheese—queso
- chili powder—chile en polvo (M), pimentón picante (S)
- chili sauce—salsa de chile (M), guindillas (S)
- chive—cebolleta
- condensed milk—leche condensada

- bouillon, beef/chicken—consomé de res (M), de carne (S) o de pollo
- broth, beef/chicken—caldo de res (M), de carne (S) o de pollo
- canned fish—pescado enlatado
- canned meat—carne enlatada
- canned tomatoes—tomates (S), jitomates (M) enlatados
- canned vegetables—verduras enlatadas
- capers—alcaparras
- catsup—salsa de tomate condimentada
- cured meats—fiambres
- garlic salt—sal de ajo
- gravy—salsa
- horseradish—raíz fuerte (M)
- instant or frozen potatoes—papas (M), patatas (S) instantaneas o congeladas
- Knorr Swiss—Knorr Suiza
- margarine—margarina
- mayonnaise—mayonesa
- meat sauce—salsa de carne
- milk—leche
- monosodium glutamate (MSG)—ajinomoto o monosodio de glutamato
- mustard—mostaza
- relish—encurtidos (M), pepinillos (S)
- Rosa Blanca
- salt—sal
- salted butter—mantequilla salada
- salted salad dressing—aderezo con sal
- sausage—productos de salchichonería
- seasoned salt—sal condimentada
- sodium preservatives—preservativos de sodio
- soy sauce—salsa de soya (M), soja (S)
- tomato puree—puré de tomate
- tomato sauce—salsa de tomate

# The Low-Sodium (Low-Salt) Scenario

If you can't pronounce the Spanish, point to appropriate phrases. For some sample replies to your questions, turn to *Appendix 1: Spanish Food Preparation* and show it to your respondent.

- **I have a reservation. My name is _____.**

Tengo reservaciones, soy el señor/la señora/la señorita _____.

- **Please tell the manager I am here.**

Por favor dígale al gerente.

■ **The manager knows about the special service I need because of a medical problem.**
El sabe del servicio especial que voy a requerir a causa de un estado de salud precaria.

■ **Does anyone here speak English?**
¿Hay álguien aquí que hable inglés?

■ **I/she/he must follow a special diet.**
Yo debo él/ella debe seguir una dieta rígida.

■ **All my/his/her food and drink must be completely salt-free.**
Toda mi/su comida debe prepararse totalmente sin sal.

■ **Everything must be prepared without the items on this list.**
Todo debe ser preparado sin los ingredientes mencionados en la lista.

■ **A mistake can cause serious illness.**
Un error podría causarme/causarle graves daños.

■ **Does this dish contain any salt?**
¿Este platillo contiene sal?

■ **Does this dish contain anything on this list?**
¿Este platillo contiéne algún ingrediente de la lista?

■ **Can you prepare this dish without salt?**
¿Le sería posible preparar este platillo sin sal?

■ **Can you prepare this dish without any of the items on this list?**
¿Podría usted preparar este platillo sin ninguno de los ingredientes mencionados en esta lista?

■ **Show me on the menu which dishes you can prepare without salt.**

Por favor, enséñeme cuáles platillos del menú se pueden preparar sin sal.

■ **Show me on the menu which dishes you can prepare without any of the items on this list.**

Por favor, enséñeme cuáles platillos del menú se pueden preparar sin ninguno de los ingredientes de la lista.

■ **Which dishes on the menu are salt-free?**

¿Cuáles platillos del menú no contienen sal?

■ **Is there any dish on the menu that does not contain ingredients forbidden to me?**

¿Hay algún platillo del menú que no contenga los ingredientes que se me han prohibido?

■ **Are the tomatoes in this dish fresh, frozen or canned? (Waiter, please point to the right word.)**

¿Los jitomates (M), tomates (S) de este platillo, son frescos, congelados o enlatados? (Mesero (M), Camarero (S), por favor muéstreme la palabra correcta.)

■ **Is the pasta cooked in salted water?**

¿Los fideos/la pasta italiana/el espagueti, se hirvieron en agua salada?

■ **Can you prepare a serving of pasta for me, cooked in unsalted water?**

¿Le sería posible prepararme una porción de fideos/ pasta italiana/el espagueti sin hervirlos en agua salada?

■ **Are the potatoes/vegetables cooked in salted water?**

¿Las papas (M), patatas (S)/verduras, se hirvieron en agua salada?

- **Can you prepare potatoes/vegetables for me, cooked in unsalted water?**

¿Le sería posible preparar las papas (M), patatas (S)/ verduras sin hervirlas en agua salada?

- **Do you prepare the tortillas in your own kitchen? With salt? With wheat flour?***

Las tortillas (M), ¿Las prepararon ustedes? ¿Con sal? ¿Con harina de trigo?

- **If you are not sure, please tell me/ask the chef/the maitre d'.**

Si no está usted seguro, por favor dígame/pregúntele al chef/pregúntele al maitre.

- **I would like to speak to the chef/the maitre d'.**

Quisiera hablar con el chef/el maitre.

- **Can you prepare something simple for me in your kitchen that is salt-free? For example, baked or broiled fish; steak; baked, boiled, or mashed potatoes; fresh, cooked, unsalted vegetables? Potatoes and vegetables must not be cooked in salted water.**

¿Le sería posible prepararme un platillo sencillo sin sal? Por ejemplo, un pescado asado o a la parrilla; un bistec; unas papas (M), patatas (S), al horno o hervidas; puré de papas (M), patatas (S), verduras frescas cocidas. Las papas (M), patatas (S) y las verduras no se deben hervir en agua salada.

- **Do you have a microwave oven/a pressure cooker?**

¿Aquí tienen un horno micro-hondas/una olla exprés?

(If the answer is *yes,* then ask:)

- **Can you prepare a single portion of _____ plain/without seasoning/gravy/sauce/salt?**

¿Le sería posible preparar una porción de _____ sencilla/sin condimentos/salsa/sal?

*Wheat flour tortillas in Mexico (mostly in the north) usually contain salt. Cornmeal tortillas are less likely to have added salt. Ask!

■ **A mistake has been made. This is not what I ordered.**
Esto es un error. No es lo que pedí.

# The Diabetic Diet

Your physician has outlined a personal diet and probably shown you how to select balanced meals using a system of food exchanges. The phrases in this section will help you identify dishes containing sweeteners on a menu. If you must also observe a low-fat diet, refer to the low-fat and low-cholesterol phrases on pages 83–86.
**Caution:** If you must take an antacid, be sure to read the information on page 15 about the sugar content of many popular antacids.

To make sure your food is properly prepared, consult *Appendix 1: Spanish Food Preparation.* Use it together with other appropriate pages when ordering meals.

Check the "not permitted" list. To make it easier for others to read, cross out the items that do not apply to you, and add things you cannot have. PRINT LEGIBLY! Select your additions from the food lists on pages 48–72.

## Foods Not Permitted – Alimentos Prohibidos

- butter—mantequilla
- condensed milk—leche condensada
- corn sweetener— endulzantes de maíz
- corn syrup—miel Karo de maíz (M)
- dextrose—dextrosa
- fats—grasa
- fructose—fructosa
- honey—miel de abeja
- jam—mermelada
- jelly—jalea
- lard—manteca
- maltose—maltosa
- margarine—margarina
- (orange) marmalade— mermelada de naranja
- molasses—melasa o piloncillo (M), azúcar morena (S)
- oils—aceite
- rice syrup—miel de arroz
- shortening—manteca vegetal
- sugar—azúcar
- syrup—miel

# The Diabetic Scenario

If you cannot pronounce the Spanish, point to the appropriate phrases. For some sample replies to your questions, turn to *Appendix 1: Spanish Food Preparation* and show it to your respondent.

■ **I have a reservation. My name is _____.**
Tengo reservaciones. Soy el señor/la señora/la señorita _____.

■ **Please tell the manager I am here.**
Por favor dígale al gerente.

■ **The manager knows about the special service I need because of a medical problem.**
El sabe que voy a requerir un servicio especial a causa de un estado de salud precaria.

■ **Does anyone here speak English?**
¿Hay álguien aquí que hable inglés?

■ **I/she/he must follow a special diet because of diabetes.**
Yo debo él/ella debe seguir una dieta muy rígida porque tengo/tiene diabetis.

■ **All food and drink must be free of added sugar or any kind of sweetening.**
Ningún alimento o bebida puede contener azúcar o endulzante de cualquier tipo.

■ **Everything must be prepared without the ingredients on this list.**
Todo se tiene que preparar sin los ingredientes mencionados en esta lista.

■ **A mistake can cause serious illness.**
Un error podría causarme/causarle graves daños.

- **Does this dish/beverage/juice contain any of the sweeteners on the list?**
¿Este platillo/esta bebida/este jugo, contiéne alguno de los endulzantes de la lista?

- **Can you prepare this dish/juice/beverage without sweetening?**
¿Le sería posible preparar este platillo/este jugo/ esta bebida sin endulzante?

- **Are the fruits/vegetables in this dish fresh/canned/frozen?**
¿Las frutas/verduras de este platillo, son frescas/ enlatadas/congeladas?

- **If it is canned or frozen in syrup, please drain all the liquid.**
Si son enlatadas o congeladas, por favor quíteles todo el líquido.

- **Do you have any artificial sweetener?**
¿Tiene usted algún endulzante artificial?

- **If you are not sure, please tell me/ask the chef/the maitre d'.**
Si no está usted seguro, por favor dígame/pregúntele al chef/pregúntele al maitre.

- **I would like to speak to the chef/the maitre d'.**
Quisiera hablar con el chef/el maitre.

- **Do you have a microwave oven/pressure cooker?**
¿Aquí tienen un horno micro-hondas/una olla exprés?

(If the answer is *yes*, then ask:)

- **Can you prepare a single portion of _____ plain/without seasoning/gravy/sauce/sugar/sweetening?**
¿Le sería posible preparar una porción de _____ sencilla/sin condimentos/salsa/azúcar/endulzante?

■ **A mistake has been made. This is not what I ordered.**
Esto es un error. No es lo que pedí.

# The Low-Fat and Low-Cholesterol Diet

The following list of "not-permitted' items may vary from the foods your physician has instructed you to avoid. To make the list easier for others to read, cross out the items that do not apply to you, and write in, PRINTING LEGIBLY, things you must avoid. Select them from the food lists on pages 48–72.

To make sure your food and drinks are prepared properly, consult *Appendix 1: Spanish Food Preparation*. Use it together with other appropriate pages when ordering meals.

Consider yourself lucky to be in Mexico or Spain where fish dishes are so popular. In both countries you can eat well and still stick to your diet if you choose fish for most of your meals. Of course, you must remember to avoid fatty sauces or fish fried in butter. Ask to have your fish served plain, unless you are sure the sauce does not have a fatty base.

## Foods Not Permitted – Alimentos Prohibidos

- all animal fats—toda grasa de animal
- all fats—grasas
- all oils—aceites
- avocado—aguacate (M)
- bacon fat—manteca de tocino
- butter—mantequilla
- canned meat/fish—carne o pescado enlatado

- cheese sauces—salsas de queso
- cheese/yogurt made from part skim or whole milk—queso/yogurt parcialmente descremado o de leche entera
- chocolate—chocolate
- cocoa—cocoa (M), cacao (S)

- cocoa butter—manteca de coco
- coconut—coco
- coconut oil—aceite de coco
- cream—crema (M), nata (S)
- eggs—huevos
- egg yolk—yema de huevo
- fried foods—alimentos fritos
- gravy—salsa
- ground meat—carne molida o picada
- heart—corazón
- hydrogenated oil—aceite hydrogenado
- kidney—riñones
- lard—manteca
- liver—hígado
- margarine—margarina
- mayonnaise—mayonesa
- nuts—nueces
- olive oil—aceite de oliva
- palm kernel oil—aceite de nuéz de palma
- palm oil—aceite de palma
- part skim milk—leche parcialmente descremada
- peanut oil—aceite de cacahuate (M), cacahuete (S)
- salad dressing oil—aderezo con aceite
- sausage—productos de salchichonería
- shortening—manteca vegetal
- shrimp—camarones (M), gambas (S)
- sour cream—crema agria
- sweetbreads—mollejas de ternera (M), lechecillas (S)
- whole milk—leche entera

# The Low-Fat and Low-Cholesterol Scenario

If you can't pronounce the Spanish, point to the appropriate phrases. For some sample replies to your questions, turn to *Appendix 1: Spanish Food Preparation* and show it to your respondent.

■ **I have a reservation. My name is _____.**

Tengo reservaciones. Soy el señor/la señora/la señorita _____.

■ **Please tell the manager I am here.**

Por favor dígale al gerente.

- **The manager knows about the special service I need because of a medical problem.**
El sabe que voy a requerir un servicio especial a causa de un estado de salud precaria.

- **Does anyone here speak English?**
¿Hay álguien aquí que hable inglés?

- **I/she/he must follow a special diet because of a serious medical problem.**
Yo debo/él/ella debe seguir una dieta rígida a causa de un serio problema médico.

- **All food and drink must be fat-free.**
Todos mis/sus alimentos y bebidas tienen que ser desgrasados.

- **Everything must be prepared without the ingredients on this list.**
Todo tiene que ser preparado sin los ingredientes de esta lista.

- **Nothing can be fried.**
No se debe freír nada.

- **All visible fat must be trimmed before cooking.**
A mis/sus alimentos se les necesita quitar toda la grasa visible antes de cocinarlos.

- **A mistake can cause serious illness.**
Un error podría causarme/causarle graves daños.

- **Does this dish contain any _____?**
¿Este platillo, contiéne _____?

- **Can you prepare this dish without _____?**
¿Le sería posible preparar este platillo sin _____?

■ **Can you prepare this dish with _____ instead of _____?**

¿Le sería posible preparar este platillo con _____ en vez de _____?

■ **Can you bake/broil this fish without sauce?**

¿Le sería posible asar/cocinar a la parrilla este pescado sin salsa?

■ **Does this dish contain anything on this list?**

¿Este platillo, contiéne alguno de los ingredientes de esta lista?

■ **Can you prepare this dish without any of the items on this list?**

¿Le sería posible preparar este platillo sin ninguno de los ingredientes de esta lista?

■ **Are there any dishes on your menu that do not contain ingredients forbidden to me?**

¿Hay algún platillo del menú que no contiene los ingredientes que se me/le prohiben?

■ **Can you fry/prepare this dish with any of these oils: safflower/sunflower/corn/soy/cottonseed/peanut?**

¿Le sería posible freír/preparar este platillo con uno de estos aceites: cártamo/girasol/maíz/soya (M), soja (S)/semilla de algodón/cacahuate (M), cacahuete (S)?

■ **Please serve this plain, without any sauce/gravy.**

Quiero este platillo muy sencillo, sin salsa.

■ **If you are not sure, please tell me/ask the chef/the maitre d'.**

Si no está usted seguro, por favor dígame/pregúntele al chef/al maitre.

■ **I would like to speak to the chef/the maitre d'.**

Quisiera hablar con el chef/el maitre.

■ **Do you have a microwave oven/a pressure cooker?**
¿Aquí tienen un horno micro-hondas/una olla exprés?

(If the answer is *yes,* then ask:)

■ **Can you prepare a single portion of _____, plain/without seasoning/gravy/sauce/butter/oil/fats?**
¿Le sería posible preparar una porción de _____ sencilla/sin condimentos/salsa/mantequilla/aceites/ grasas?

■ **A mistake has been made. This is not what I ordered.**
Esto es un error. No es lo que pedí.

# The Ulcer, Bland, Soft, and Low-Residue Diet

The items on the following list may vary from the foods your physician has instructed you to avoid. To make the list easier for others to read, cross out the items that do not apply to you, and add, PRINTING LEGIBLY, the things you cannot have. Select them from the food lists on pages 48–72.

To make sure your food and drink are prepared properly, consult *Appendix 1: Spanish Food Preparation.* Use it together with other appropriate pages when ordering meals.

You are probably aware of the highly seasoned dishes in Mexican cuisine. Although Spain's dishes are not quite as "hot," you must still be careful; many have enough seasoning in them to wreck a sensitive digestive system. As a result, your best bet is to stay with dishes that can be prepared directly to your order. Broiled or baked fish are excellent choices. Meat dishes, such as broiled chops or steaks, are also easy for the chef to tailor to your needs.

# Foods Not Permitted – Alimentos Prohibidos

- bran—salvado
- brown rice—arroz integral
- catsup—salsa de jitomate (M), tomate (S) condimentada
- chili—chile (M), guindillas (S)
- clams—almejas
- coarse bread—pan integral
- coarse cereals—cereales integrales
- coconut—coco
- corn—maíz
- dried fruits—frutas secas
- dried legumes—todo tipo de leguminosas secas
- fat—grasa
- foods prepared with wine or liqueurs—alimentos preparados con vino o licores
- fried foods—alimentos fritos
- garlic—ajo
- gravy—salsa
- herbs—hierbas de olor
- horseradish—raíz fuerte (M)
- lard—manteca
- meat broth—caldo de carne
- mustard—mostaza
- nuts/seeds—nueces o semillas
- olives—aceitunas
- onions—cebolla
- oysters—ostiones (M), ostras (S)
- paprika—paprika (M), pimentón (S)
- peas—chícharos (M), guisantes (S)
- pepper—pimienta
- pickled meat/fish—carne o pescado encurtido (M), en vinagre (S)
- pork—carne de cerdo
- raisins—pasas
- relish—encurtidos (M), pepinillos (S)
- salt—sal
- sauce—salsas
- seasoning—condimentos
- sharp (strong) cheese—quesos fuertes
- spices—especias
- vinegar—vinagre

# The Ulcer, Bland, Soft, and Low-Residue Scenario

If you cannot pronounce the Spanish, point to appropriate phrases. For some sample replies to your questions, turn to *Appendix 1: Spanish Food Preparation* and show it to your respondent.

- **I have a reservation. My name is _____.**
Tengo reservaciones. Soy el señor/la señora/la señorita _____.

- **Please tell the manager I am here.**
  Por favor dígale al gerente.

- **The manager knows about the special service I need because of a medical problem.**
  El sabe que voy a requerir un servicio especial a causa de un estado de salud precaria.

- **Does anyone here speak English?**
  ¿Hay álguien aquí que hable inglés?

- **I/she/he must follow a special diet for a stomach problem.**
  Yo debo/él/ella debe seguir una dieta rígida por un problema estomacal.

- **Everything must be prepared without spices/seasoning.**
  Todo tiene que ser preparado sin especias o condimentos.

- **Nothing can be fried. Food must be baked/broiled/stewed/ poached.**
  No se debe freir nada. Mis/sus alimentos tienen que ser asados/a la parrilla/hervidos o estofados.

- **A mistake can cause serious illness.**
  Un error podría causarme/causarle graves daños.

- **Please bake/broil/stew/poach this dish.**
  Haga el favor de estofar/hervir a la parrilla/hervir/ estofar este platillo.

- **Can you bake/broil/stew/poach this dish?**
  ¿Le sería posible asar/cocinar a la parrilla/estofar/ hervir este platillo?

- **Everything must be prepared without the ingredients on this list. Please read it. Thank you.**

Todo tiene que ser preparado sin los ingredientes de esta lista. Por favor léala. Gracias.

- **Does this dish contain any _____?**

¿Este platillo contiéne _____?

- **Can you prepare this dish without _____?**

¿Le sería posible preparar este platillo sin _____?

- **Can you prepare this dish with _____ instead of _____?**

¿Le sería posible preparar este platillo con _____ en vez de _____?

- **If you are not sure, please tell me/ask the chef/the maitre d'.**

Si no está usted seguro, por favor dígame/pregúntele al chef/pregúntele al maitre.

- **Can you prepare something bland and simple like a platter of plain baked fish, baked potato or plain boiled potatoes, tender carrots or spinach or green beans or mushrooms?**

¿Le sería posible preparar algo muy sencillo como un platillo de pescado asado sin condimentos, unas papas (M), patatas (S) asadas o hervidas, zanahorias muy tiernas o espinacas o ejotes (M), judías verdes (S) o hongos (M), setas (S)?

- **Do you have a microwave oven/pressure cooker?**

¿Aquí tienen un horno micro-hondas/una olla exprés?

(If the answer is *yes,* then ask:)

- **Can you prepare a single portion of _____, plain/without seasoning/gravy/sauce?**

¿Le sería posible prepararme una porción de _____ sencilla/sin condimentos/salsa?

■ **A mistake has been made. This is not what I ordered.**
Esto es un error. No es lo que pedí.

■ **I would like to speak to the chef/the maitre d'.**
Quisiera hablar con el chef/el maitre.

# Design Your Own Scenario for a Custom-made Diet

If, for health, personal or religious reasons, you require a special diet that does not appear in this repertoire, you can produce your own script. We've made it easy for you by supplying the phrases on the following pages. To fill in the blanks of phrases you plan to use, do the following:

**1.** On a separate sheet of paper, prepare a list of foods you cannot eat.

**2.** Translate them into Spanish, using the "not permitted" lists of the other diets and the food lists on pages 48–72; you may also find the supplementary lists at the end of this chapter useful.

**3.** Copy the list into this book, PRINTING LEGIBLY in the blank spaces provided under the heading "not permitted." PRINT it in English *and* Spanish.

**4.** PRINT the Spanish words, where applicable, in the blanks in the script.

**5.** Don't forget to use *Appendix 1: Spanish Food Preparation* to explain how you want your food prepared.

| Foods Not Permitted | Alimentos Prohibidos |
|---|---|
|  |  |
|  |  |
|  |  |
|  |  |
|  |  |
|  |  |

| Foods Not Permitted | Alimentos Prohibidos |
|---|---|
| _____ | _____ |
| _____ | _____ |
| _____ | _____ |
| _____ | _____ |
| _____ | _____ |
| _____ | _____ |
| _____ | _____ |
| _____ | _____ |

# The Custom-made Scenario

If you can't pronounce the Spanish, point to appropriate phrases. For some sample replies to your questions, turn to *Appendix 1: Spanish Food Preparation* and show it to your respondent.

■ **I have a reservation. My name is _____.**
Tengo reservaciones. Soy el señor/la señora/la señorita _____.

■ **Please tell the manager I am here.**
Por favor dígale al gerente.

■ **The manager knows about the special service I need because of a medical problem.**
El sabe que voy a requerir un servicio especial a causa de un estado de salud precaria.

■ **The manager knows about the special diet I need.**
El gerente sabe que voy a requerir una dieta especial.

■ **Does anyone here speak English?**
¿Hay álguien aquí que hable inglés?

■ **I/she/he must follow a special diet.**
Yo debo/él/ella debe seguir una dieta especial.

■ **All my/his/her food and drink must be prepared without**
_____.
Mi/su comida y mis/sus bebidas necesitan prepararse sin nada de _____.

■ **Everything must be prepared without the items on this list.**
Todo se tiene que preparar sin los alimentos indicados en esta lista.

■ **A mistake can cause serious illness.**
Un error podría causarme/causarle una grave
enfermedad.

■ **Does this dish contain any _____?**
¿Este platillo contiene _____?

■ **Does this dish contain anything on this list?**
¿Este platillo, contiene alguno de los alimentos
mencionados en la lista?

■ **Can you prepare this dish without _____?**
¿Le sería posible preparar este platillo sin _____?

■ **Show me on the menu which dishes you can prepare without**
_____.
Enséñeme cuáles platillos del menú se podrían
preparar sin _____.

■ **Show me on the menu which dishes you can prepare without
any of the items on this list.**
Enséñeme cuáles platillos del menú se podrían
preparar sin ninguno de los alimentos indicados en
la lista.

- **Are there any dishes on the menu that do not contain ingredients forbidden to me?**
¿Hay algún platillo del menú que no contenga los ingredientes que se me prohiben?

- **If you are not sure, please tell me/ask the chef/the maitre d'.**
Si no está usted seguro, por favor dígame/pregúntele al chef/pregúntele al maitre.

- **I would like to speak to the chef/the maitre d'.**
Quisiera hablar con el chef/el maitre.

- **Can you prepare something simple for me in your kitchen that is appropriate for my diet? For example: _____.**
¿Le sería posible prepararme algo muy sencillo apropiado para mi dieta? Por ejemplo: _____.

- **Do you have a microwave oven/a pressure cooker?**
¿Tienen ustedes un horno micro-hondas/una olla exprés?

(If the answer is *yes*, then ask:)

- **Can you prepare a single portion of _____ without _____?**
¿Le sería posible prepararme una porción de _____ sin _____?

- **A mistake has been made. This is not what I ordered.**
Esto es un error. No es lo que pedí.

To compose a list of forbidden items, consult the food lists on pages 48–72, the collection of no-nos for the other scenarios, and this sampling of foods that can cause reactions in some allergenic and otherwise sensitive individuals.

# Possible Forbidden Items – Alimentos Prohibidos

- barley–cebada perla
- barley cereal–cereal de cebada perla
- barley flour–harina de cebada perla
- beef–carne de res (M), vaca (S)
- beets–betabel (M), remolacha (S)
- bran–salvado
- buckwheat–trigo negro
- buckwheat cereal–cereal de trigo negro
- buckwheat flour–harina de trigo negro
- buckwheat stuffing–relleno de trigo negro
- chocolate–chocolate
- cinnamon–canela
- citrus fruits–limones, limas, naranjas, toronjas, mandarinas
- coconut–coco
- coffee–café
- cola–productos con cola
- corn–maíz
- corn products–productos de maíz
- dates–dátiles
- eggs–huevos
- figs–higos
- fish–pescado
- flax seeds–semillas de lino
- legumes–todo frijol (M), judías secas (S); chícharo (M), guisante (S); lenteja o garbanzo seco
- lettuce–lechuga
- malt–malta
- malt flavoring–sabor de malta
- milk–leche
- nuts–nueces

- oat flour–harina de avena
- oatmeal bread–pan de avena
- oatmeal cereal–cereal de avena
- oatmeal stuffing–relleno de avena
- oats–avena
- peanuts–cacahuates (M), cacahuetes (S)
- pork–carne de cerdo
- potato–papa (M), patata (S)
- rice–arroz
- ripe beans–todo tipo de leguminosas frescas
- rye–centeno
- rye bread–pan de centeno
- rye bread crumbs–pan molido de centeno
- rye cereal–cereal de centeno
- rye flour–harina de centeno
- shellfish–mariscos
- soybeans–soya (M), soja (S)
- string beans–ejotes (M), judías verdes (S)
- tomato–jitomate (M), tomate (S)
- wheat–trigo
- wheat bread–pan de trigo
- wheat bread crumbs–pan molido de trigo
- wheat cereal–cereal de trigo
- wheat flour–harina de trigo
- wheat germ–germen de trigo
- wheat germ oil–aceite de germen de trigo
- wheat stuffing–relleno de trigo
- yeast–levadura

# Medical Aid

Read these pages now. They will make things easier for you later.

In an acute emergency ask a Spanish-speaking person to telephone for help for you. You will find the phrase for such a request under *Emergencies* on page 97. Memorize it now.

## U.S. Embassy and Consular Assistance in Mexico

If you are visiting Mexico City, you can obtain a list of qualified English-speaking physicians from the American Embassy. It's a good thing to keep handy. Why wait for an emergency? Get your umbrella before it rains! So, when in Mexico, drop in for the list at the:

**Embassy of the United States** — Paseo de la Reforma 305, Mexico City D. F. Telephone: 905-553-3333.

Consular services are available in other Mexican cities, too:

**Ciudad Juárez** — 924 Avenida Lopez Mateos, Ciudad Juárez, Chihuahua. Telephone: 34048.

**Guadalajara** — Progreso 175, Guadalajara, Jalisco. Telephone: 25-29-98 or 25-27-00.

**Hermosillo** — Isssteson Building, 3rd floor, Miguel Hidalgo Y Costilla No. 15, Hermosillo, Sonora. Telephone: 3-89-22/23/24.

**Matamoros** — Avenida Primera No. 232, Matamoros, Tamaulipas. Telephone: 2-52-50/51/52.

**Mazatlán** — 6 Circunvalación No. 6 (at Venustiano Carranza), Mazatlán, Sinaloa. Telephone: 1-29-05.

**Mérida** — Paseo Montejo 453, Apartado Postal 130, Mérida, Yucatán. Telephone: 7-70-78/11.

**Monterrey** — Avenida Constitución 411 Poniente, Monterrey, Nuevo León. Telephone: 4306 50/59.

**Nuevo Laredo** — Avenida Allende 3330, Col. Jardín, Nuevo Laredo, Tamaulipas. Telephone: 4-05-12 or 4-06-18.

**Tijuana** — Tapachula 96, Tijuana, Baja California Norte. Telephone: 6-1001.

# U.S. Embassy and Consular Assistance in Spain

If you're on the other side of the Atlantic Ocean, in Madrid or in three other Spanish cities, you can get lists of qualified, English-speaking physicians at the embassy and these consulate offices:

**The Embassy of the United States** — Serrano 75, Madrid. Telephone: 276-3400/3600.

Consulate service is available in these Spanish cities:

**Barcelona** — Via Layetana 33. Telephone: 319-9550.

**Bilbao** — Avenida del Ejercito 11, 3rd floor, Deusto-Bilbao 12. Telephone: 435-8308/9.

**Sevilla** — Paseo de las Delicias No. 7. Telephone: 23-1885.

# Emergencies

■ **Help!**
  ¡Auxilio!

■ **Police!**
  ¡Policía!

■ **Fire!**
  ¡Incendio!

■ **I am ill.**
  Estoy enfermo(a).

■ **She is ill.**
  Está enferma.

- **He is ill.**
  Está enfermo.

- **Call a doctor right away.**
  Llame a un médico inmediatamente.

- **Call an ambulance right away.**
  Llame una ambulancia inmediatamente.

- **Take me/us to a doctor right away.**
  Lléveme/llévenos con un médico inmediatamente.

- **Take me/us to a hospital right away.**
  Lléveme/llévenos al hospital inmediatamente.

- **Is there a doctor in the building?**
  ¿Hay un doctor en este edificio?

- **I cannot speak Spanish. Please call this number for me.**
  No sé hablar español. Por favor hable a este número de mi parte.

# Emergency Telephone Numbers

When you arrive at your lodgings and check in, ask the clerk or manager to supply you with emergency numbers. Of course, you'll feel silly making such a request before you've even seen your room or unpacked your bags. But no matter. Try out these phrases, and when you've got the numbers, fill in the blanks of the *Emergency Telephone Numbers* box that follows. Or better still, ask the clerk to fill it in for you. If you show him or her the book with this official-looking box, your request won't appear so strange.

- **Emergency numbers belong in this box. Would you mind filling it in for me? Thank you.**
  Por favor, hágame el favor de escribir los teléfonos de emergencia en este espacio. Gracias.

---

**Emergency Telephone Numbers—
Teléfonos de Emergencia**

Ambulance—Ambulancia: _____

Fire—Incendio: _____

Police—Policía: _____

---

# Asking for Help

- **Where is the nearest doctor?**
  ¿En dónde puedo localizar el médico más cercano?

- **Where is the nearest hospital/clinic?**
  ¿Dónde está el hospital/la clínica más cercano/a?

- **Where is the nearest first-aid station?**
  ¿Dónde está la clínica de primeros auxilios más cercana?

- **Where is the nearest pharmacy?**
  ¿Dónde está la farmacia más cercana?

- **Where is the nearest English-speaking doctor?**
  ¿Dónde puedo localizar el médico más cercano que hable inglés?

- **Is there an English-speaking doctor here?**
  ¿Hay un médico que hable inglés aquí?

■ **Is there a hospital here with English-speaking doctors?**
¿Hay aquí un hospital con médicos que hablen inglés?

■ **At what time can the doctor come?**
¿A qué hora puede venir el doctor?

■ **What are the office hours?**
¿Cúal es su horario de oficina?

■ **Please PRINT the information. Thank you.**
Por favor escriba la información EN LETRA DE MOLDE. Gracias.

■ **What is the doctor's name, address, and telephone number?**
¿Cómo se llama el doctor? ¿Cuál es su dirección y su número de teléfono?

■ **Please show me where it is on this map.**
Por favor enséñeme en este mapa en dónde queda.

■ **Please show me on the map where we are now.**
Por favor enséñeme en el mapa en dónde estamos ahora.

■ **Please draw a map/sketch for me.**
Por favor hágame un mapa/un dibujo.

■ **I cannot speak Spanish. Please phone for me.**
No sé hablar español. Por favor hable por teléfono de mi parte.

■ **Does anyone here speak English?**
¿Hay álguien aquí que hable inglés?

■ **I need an interpreter.**
Necesito un intérprete.

# Numbers

| | |
|---|---|
| 0 — cero | 31 — treinta y un(o) |
| 1 — uno, una, un | 32 — treinta y dos |
| 2 — dos | 40 — cuarenta |
| 3 — tres | 41 — cuarenta y un(o) |
| 4 — cuatro | 42 — cuarenta y dos |
| 5 — cinco | 50 — cincuenta |
| 6 — seis | 51 — cincuenta y un(o) |
| 7 — siete | 52 — cincuenta y dos |
| 8 — ocho | 60 — sesenta |
| 9 — nueve | 61 — sesenta y un(o) |
| 10 — diez | 62 — sesenta y dos |
| 11 — once | 70 — setenta |
| 12 — doce | 80 — ochenta |
| 13 — trece | 90 — noventa |
| 14 — catorce | 100 — cien |
| 15 — quince | 101 — ciento un(o) |
| 16 — dieciséis | 102 — ciento dos |
| 17 — diecisiete | 200 — doscientos, -as |
| 18 — dieciocho | 300 — trescientos, -as |
| 19 — diecinueve | 500 — quinientos, -as |
| 20 — veinte | 1000 — mil |
| 21 — veintiuno, veintiún | half — medio(a) |
| 22 — veintidós | quarter — un cuarto |
| 30 — treinta | |

# Section Three:
# Say It in German

# German Pronunciation

German pronunciation is relatively uncomplicated once you have mastered a few changes in vowel sounds and in those of certain consonants. Each German word is pronounced separately; the words do not run together as sentences are spoken.

## Vowels

German vowels can be long or short. As a rule, they are short in unaccented syllables or when followed by two or more consonants. Vowels are long when they are doubled or followed by an H.

| | Long | Short |
|---|---|---|
| A | as in FATHER | as in CUT |
| E | similar to CAFÉ | as in GET |
| I | as in MACHINE | as in HIT |
| O | rounder than HOLE | similar to OFTEN |
| U | as in LOOT | as in PUT |
| ä | as in FARE | as in GET |
| ö | pronounce long E as in CAFÉ with lips rounded | pronounce short E as in GET with lips rounded |
| ü | pronounce long I as in MACHINE with lips rounded and protruded | pronounce short I as in BIT with lips rounded and protruded |
| Y | sometimes pronounced ü; sometimes like short I | |

## Diphthongs

**AU**   as in HOUSE
**EI, AI, AY,** and **EY**   as in LIKE
**EU, AU**   as in COIN

102

# Consonants

Only those consonants that are *not* pronounced as they are in English are mentioned here.

**B, D, G** in the final position of a word are pronounced P, T, K, respectively

**J** pronounced like **Y**ES

**R** —no English equivalent; but an English R will be understood

**S** before vowels is similar to Z; otherwise like **S** in **S**EE

**SS** pronounced sharp as **S** in **S**EE

**V** pronounced like **F** in **F**ATHER (but in words of foreign origin, pronounced like **V** in English: as in UNI**V**ERSITÄT)

**W** as in **V**ERY

**Z** as **TS** in NU**TS**

**CH** —no English equivalent, but similar to **CH** in the Scottish LO**CH**. When it is the first letter of a word and is followed by A, O, or a consonant, it is pronounced as a **K**.

**CHS** pronounced KS

**CK** pronounced like K

**DT** pronounced like T

**GN, KN, PF, PS** —both consonants of each set pronounced

**PH** pronounced like F

**QU** pronounced like KV

**SCH** pronounced like **SH** in **SH**E

**SP** pronounced SHP when it opens a syllable; pronounced SP in other positions

**ST** pronounced SHT when it opens a syllable; pronounced ST in other positions

**TH** pronounced T

**TZ** pronounced like **TS** in NU**TS**

German

Pronunciation

# Basic Expressions in German

- **Yes**
  Ja

- **No**
  Nein

- **Hello**
  Guten Tag

- **Please**
  Bitte

- **Thank you**
  Danke

- **Excuse me**
  Entschuldigung

- **Pardon me**
  Verzeihung

- **Good morning, Good afternoon, Good evening**
  Guten Morgen, Guten Tag, Guten Abend

- **Good night, Good-bye**
  Gute Nacht, Auf Wiedersehen

- **Where is the ladies'/men's room?**
  Wo ist die Damen/Herren Toilette?

- **My name is _____.**
  Mein Name ist _____.

- **I am staying at _____.**
  Ich wohne im _____.

- **Can you help me?**
  Können Sie mir helfen?

- **Do you speak English?**
  Sprechen Sie Englisch?

- **Does anyone here speak English?**
  Spricht hier jemand Englisch?

- **Can you find someone who speaks English?**
  Können Sie jemanden finden, der Englisch spricht?

- **I do not understand that.**
  Ich verstehe das nicht.

- **Please speak slowly.**
  Bitte sprechen Sie langsam.

- **Please repeat it.**
  Bitte wiederholen Sie das.

- **Please PRINT the directions.**
  Bitte *drucken* Sie die Weganweisung.

- **Please PRINT it. Please write it down.**
  Bitte *drucken* Sie es. Bitte schreiben Sie es auf.

- **Please PRINT the name, address, and telephone number.**
  Bitte *drucken* Sie den Namen, die Adresse, und die Telefonnummer.

Basic Expressions

- **Please show me on this map.**
Bitte zeigen Sie es mir auf dieser Karte.

- **Please show me on this map where I am.**
Bitte zeigen Sie mir auf dieser Karte, wo ich bin.

- **Please draw a map/sketch for me.**
Bitte zeichnen Sie es für mich auf.

- **Please call this number for me. Thank you.**
Bitte rufen Sie diese Nummer für mich an. Vielen Dank.

- **Where is the nearest _____?**
Wo ist das (der, die) nächste _____?
    - **hospital/clinic**
    Krankenhaus/Klinik
    - **first aid facility**
    Erste Hilfe Station
    - **diet/health food/natural food restaurant**
    Restaurant mit Diät Essen

- **Is the restaurant open/closed now?**
Ist das Restaurant jetzt offen/geschlossen?

- **Please point to the days and hours it is open/closed.**
Bitte zeigen Sie auf die Wochentage und Stunden an denen es offen/geschlossen ist.

- **Monday**
Montag

- **Tuesday**
Dienstag

- **Wednesday**
  Mittwoch

- **Thursday**
  Donnerstag

- **Friday**
  Freitag

- **Saturday**
  Samstag or Sonnabend

- **Sunday**
  Sonntag

- **a quarter past**
  Viertel nach

- **half past (actually half of the following hour)**
  Halb

- **a quarter to**
  Viertel vor

- **morning**
  Morgens

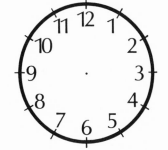

- **afternoon**
  Nachmittags

- **evening**
  Abends

- **How much is this? Please write it down. (For a list of numbers, see page 160.)**

  Wieviel kostet das? Bitte schreiben Sie es auf.

- **Do you have _____?**
  Haben Sie _____?

- **I would like _____.**
  Ich möchte bitte _____.

- **Please give me _____.**
  Bitte geben Sie mir _____.

# Dining Out in Germany

This section is divided into three parts. Part 1 includes a description of the hours for mealtimes, the available types of eating establishments, tipping customs, plus some techniques of finding a restaurant and making reservations. Also, after finding a restaurant, there are questions included which you may need to ask, such as how to find a smoke-free spot. Part 2 gives some basic food lists arranged in breakfast, lunch, and dinner order. Part 3 contains a series of diet scenarios, each linked to specific health problems plus a scenario adaptable to the needs of travelers on special diets not covered in the more specific scenarios. Look them over now and check those items that will come in handy later.

## Part 1

### Mealtimes in Germany

For most Germans lunch is the main meal of the day and consists of several courses. You can expect an extensive menu, but fast food and sandwiches can also be ordered. If you drop into an eating establishment during off-hours, the waiter will assume that you want only a cup of coffee or a cold drink, and so you must ask for a menu if you want more:

■ **The menu, please.**
Die Speisekarte, bitte.

In general, food is served in abundant quantities, but don't feel you must stuff yourself with all the courses offered. Skip as many as you please. Often appetizers are served in such quantity and so elaborately garnished that they can do for a main course.

Breakfast:   served between 7:00 and 10:00
Lunch:   served between 12:00 and 2:00
Dinner:   served between 6:00 and 10:00

# Types of Eating Establishments in Germany

**Bahnhofsgaststätte** — restaurant at a railroad station; open late, sometimes all night. Complete meals; also fast food and sandwiches.
**Buffet** — *(Selbstbedienungs*—self-service) restaurant or cafeteria. Many are located in supermarkets.
**Café** — coffeehouse where pastries and cakes are served. Sometimes soups and sandwiches are also available. Open until about 4:00 A.M.
**Gaststätte, Gasthaus, Gasthof** — restaurant; usually open until midnight.
**Imbissstuben, Schnellimbiss** — fast food restaurants and hot dog stands.
**Raststätte** — restaurant along the freeway (or Autobahn). Fast food, sandwiches, often full meals. The quality of food is usually low. Many are open 24 hours.

# Tipping in Germany

Tips and taxes are included in the prices on the menu. At the bottom of the menu, you usually find this inscription: *MWST und Trinkgeld in den Preisen miteinbeschlossen.* It means that tax and a tip have been added to the price listed. If it's not included, the server may automatically add 10 percent to your bill. You won't get your bill until you ask for it:

■ **The check, please.**

Die Rechnung bitte. Ich möchte zahlen.

# Making Reservations in German Restaurants

Let the chef know you're coming and that you must observe a special diet. Ask your hotel manager or desk clerk to phone ahead for you. If you don't speak German, and they don't speak English, simply point to the appropriate phrases.

Ask the desk clerk or manager to read the following section before he or she phones for a reservation. To describe your needs, fill in the blanks with words and phrases selected from the "not permitted" list under your diet, the diet's scenario, the food lists, and the food preparation information in *Appendix 2.*

■ **Can you recommend a good, but not too expensive restaurant?**

Können Sie ein gutes, preiswertes Restaurant empfehlen?

■ **I have/she/he has a special problem and would like you to read the following:**

Ich habe/sie/er hat ein besonderes Problem und ich bitte Sie, das Folgende zu lesen:

■ **I must ask a special favor of you. I have/she/he has a medical problem and must observe a very special diet.**

Ich muss Sie um einen Gefallen bitten. Ich habe/er/sie hat ein Gesundheitsproblem und muss eine strenge Diät einhalten.

■ **Since I cannot speak German, may I ask you to phone the restaurant and explain the problem?**

Da ich kein Deutsch spreche, möchte ich Sie bitten, das Restaurant für mich anzurufen und die Situation zu erklären.

- **May I ask you to do a favor for me/for us? Please phone this restaurant and make a reservation for a party of _____ for me for lunch/dinner. For today/tomorrow. For Monday/Tuesday/Wednesday/Thursday/Friday/Saturday/Sunday. At _____ o'clock.**
Könnten Sie mir/uns einen Gefallen tun? Bitte rufen Sie dieses Restaurant an und reservieren Sie einen Tisch für _____ Personen für mich/zum Mittagessen/zum Abendessen. Für heute/morgen. Für Montag/Dienstag/Mittwoch/Donnerstag/Freitag/Samstag/Sonntag. Um _____ Uhr.

- **I/she/he cannot eat anything containing _____.**
Ich/sie/er darf nichts mit _____ essen.

- **A mistake can cause serious illness.**
Ein Versehen könnte zu einer schweren Krankheit führen.

- **Ask the maitre d' if he will be so kind as to arrange for simple substitutions in the dishes served to me.**
Bitte fragen Sie den Oberkellner, ob es möglich ist, die Speise meiner Diät anzupassen.

- **For example, for lunch/dinner I would like _____ or _____.**
Zum Beispiel: zum Mittagessen/Abendessen möchte ich gern _____ oder _____.

- **It should be _____ (method of preparation – see *Appendix 2*).**
Ich hätte es gern _____ (Methode der Vorbereitung).

- **It should not contain any _____.**
Es darf kein _____ enthalten.

- **Please ask for the name of the person with whom you are speaking. Write it down (PRINT it) for me. Thank you very much.**

  Bitte erkundigen Sie sich nach dem Namen der Person, mit der Sie sprechen. Schreiben Sie es mir auf (in Druckschrift). Vielen Dank.

- **Please PRINT the name, address, and telephone number. Thank you.**

  Bitte schreiben Sie den Namen, die Adresse, und die Telefonnummer in Druckschrift auf. Vielen Dank.

After the call has been made, you can ask:

- **Have you made the reservation?**

  Haben Sie die Vorbestellung gemacht?

- **Did they understand my/her/his problem?**

  Hat man mein/sein/ihr Gesundheitsproblem verstanden?

- **Are they willing to arrange for special dishes?**

  Ist man gewillt, diese Speiseänderungen vorzunehmen?

  You'll find these phrases helpful if you choose a restaurant on the spur of the moment.

- **Are reservations necessary?**

  Muss ich einen Tisch reservieren lassen?

- **A table for _____, please. (See list of numbers on page 160.)**

  Einen Tisch für _____ Personen, bitte.

- **Do you have a nonsmoking section?**

  Haben Sie einen Raum für Nichtraucher?

- **Please, can you seat me/us as far away from smokers as possible?**
Könnten wir bitte so weit wie möglich von Rauchern entfernt sitzen?

- **I have/she/he has a serious allergy to smoke.**
Ich bin/sie, er ist/gegen Rauch sehr allergisch.

- **Where is the ladies'/men's room?**
Wo ist die Damen/Herren/Toilette?

- **Do you have _____?**
Haben Sie _____?

- **I would like _____.**
Ich möchte bitte _____.

- **Please give me _____.**
Bitte geben Sie mir _____.

   - **glass of water**
   ein Glas Wasser

   - **bottle of carbonated water sealed/unopened**
   eine Flasche Wasser mit Kohlensäure/ geschlossen

   - **bottle of mineral water**
   eine Flasche Mineralwasser

   - **fork/knife/spoon/napkin/straws**
   Gabel/Messer/Löffel/Serviette/Strohhalme

# Part 2

The phrases and food lists in this section will be a big help in restaurants, supermarkets, and food stores. For a list of numbers, see page 160.

# Breakfast

If you are staying at a hotel, a continental breakfast will most likely be included in the price of your room. Typically, a continental breakfast consists of fresh bread or rolls, butter, jam, and a beverage (usually tea or coffee). You may also ask for eggs, but you must specify how you want them prepared or you'll get them soft boiled. Some hotels offer a greater variety in these mini-breakfasts— sometimes cold cuts and cheeses and often a choice of pastries. Orange juice is not normally a part of a German breakfast, but it's usually available, so don't hesitate to ask. Chances are you'll get canned or bottled juice. Rarely is it prepared from frozen concentrate.

- **Do you have _____?**
  Haben Sie _____?

- **I would like _____.**
  Ich möchte bitte _____.

- **Please give me _____.**
  Bitte geben Sie mir _____.

## Fruit Juices — Säfte

Choose the fruit on this list and add "-saft" to the appropriate German word.

*English—German*
- apple—Apfel
- apricots—Aprikosen
- currants, black— schwarzer Johannisbeer
- currants, red—roter Johannisbeer
- grapefruits— Pampelmusen
- grapes, blue—roter Trauben

*German-English*
- Apfel—apple
- Aprikosen—apricots
- Birnen—pears
- Himbeer—red raspberries
- Orangen—oranges
- Pampelmusen— grapefruits
- roter Johannisbeer—red currants

*(continued on next page)*

German

Dining Out

# Fruit Juices – Säfte (continued)

**English – German**
- grapes, green – weisser Trauben
- lemons – Zitronen
- oranges – Orangen
- pears – Birnen
- raspberries, red – Himbeer
- tomatoes – Tomaten

**German – English**
- roter Trauben – blue grapes
- schwarzer Johannisbeer black currants
- Tomaten – tomatoes
- weisser Trauben – green grapes
- Zitronen – lemons

# Fruit – Früchte

**English – German**
- apples – Apfel
- apricots – Aprikosen
- avocado – Avokado
- bananas – Bananen
- blackberries – Brombeeren
- blueberries – Blaubeeren
- cherries – Kirschen
- cranberries – Preisselbeeren
- currants, black – schwarze Johannisbeeren
- currants, red – rote Johannisbeeren
- dates – Datteln
- figs – Feigen
- gooseberries – Stachelbeeren
- grapefruits – Pampelmusen
- grapes, blue – blaue Trauben
- grapes, green – grüne Trauben
- lemons – Zitronen
- melons – Melonen
- nuts – Nüsse

**German – English**
- Ananas – pineapples
- Äpfel – apples
- Aprikosen – apricots
- Avokado – avocado
- Bananen – bananas
- Birnen – pears
- Blaubeeren – blueberries
- Brombeeren – blackberries
- Datteln – dates
- Erdbeeren – strawberries
- Feigen – figs
- Himbeeren – raspberries
- Kirschen – cherries
- Mandarinen – tangerines
- Melonen – melons
- Nüsse – nuts
- Oliven – olives
- Orangen – oranges
- Pampelmusen – grapefruits
- Pfirsiche – peaches
- Pflaumen – plums
- Preisselbeeren – cranberries
- Rosinen – raisins

## English—German

- olives—Oliven
- oranges—Orangen
- peaches—Pfirsiche
- pears—Birnen
- pineapples—Ananas
- plums—Pflaumen
- prunes—getrocknete Pflaumen
- raisins—Rosinen
- raspberries—Himbeeren
- strawberries—Erdbeeren
- tangerines—Mandarinen
- tomatoes—Tomaten

## German-English

- rote Johannisbeeren— red currants
- schwarze Johannisbeeren— black currants
- Stachelbeeren— gooseberries
- Tomaten—tomatoes
- Trauben, blaue—blue grapes
- Trauben, grüne—green grapes
- Zitronen—lemons

Now that you've had your fruit juice and/or fruit, are you ready for something else? You should be. A hearty breakfast will keep you going for hours and stave off the hunger that often traps you into stuffing yourself at dinner. If your hotel offers only continental breakfasts and you'd like to augment it, speak with the manager or the maitre d' the day or evening before your first morning meal. Try these phrases:

- **May I ask a special favor of you?**
  Dürfte ich Sie um einen Gefallen bitten?

- **Would it be possible to have _____ for breakfast?**
  Wäre es möglich, _____ zum Frühstück zu bekommen?

Select something from the following lists of breakfast foods, but keep it simple. If necessary, show your WALLET CARD; it will lend authority to your request. If your food must be prepared in a special way, point to the appropriate phrases (Appendix 2). Better still, put it all down on paper before you approach the maitre d'. PRINT IT! Of course, you'll be a little embarrassed the first time you make a special request and flash your WALLET CARD. Who wouldn't be? But keep in mind that it's the hotel staff's job to make your stay a comfortable one. The important thing is to be polite and friendly in making your request. And remember: after you've done it once, you'll quickly become an old hand at it. Okay, let's get back to breakfast.

# Cereals – Brei

If you'd like a bowl of hot or cold cereal, try the following phrases. A whole range of cold cereals can be called either "Cornflakes" or *Getreide Flocken*. Have a look at the picture or list of ingredients on the container before digging in.

■ **Please cook it in unsalted water.**
Bitte kochen Sie es in ungesalzenem Wasser.

■ **Don't put any _____ in it.**
Fügen Sie bitte kein _____ hinzu.

■ **Please put some _____ in it.**
Geben Sie bitte etwas _____ hinzu.

■ **Do you have _____?**
Haben Sie _____?

■ **I would like _____.**
Ich möchte bitte _____.

■ **Please give me _____.**
Bitte geben Sie mir _____.

The following cereals are sometimes available in restaurants:
• barley—Graupen
• barley, pearl—Gerstengrütze
• bran—Kleie
• buckwheat—Buchweizen
• cornmeal—Maisschleim/Maisbrei
• farina—Griessbrei
• groats—Hafergrütze
• gruel—Haferschleim
• millet—Hirse
• oat flakes, coarse—Haferflocken

- oatmeal, fine—Haferbrei
- rice, brown—brauner Reis
- rice, white—weisser Reis
- rice pudding (warm)—Reisbrei
- soy—soja
- wheat germ—Weizenkeime
- whole wheat flakes—Weizenflocken

If your digestive problem requires a highly refined cereal, ask:

■ **Do you have any highly refined cereal suitable for babies?**
Haben Sie irgendwelchen feinen Brei, wie zum Beispiel für Babys?

# Bread, Rolls, and Pancakes—
# Brot, Brötchen, und Pfannkuchen

There are a great many kinds of bread in Germany, because tastes differ from region to region. Here are some staple types that you can find almost anywhere:
- Brötchen—hard rolls
- Knäckebrot—a flat bread, low in calories; comes salted or unsalted (salzlos)
- Kommissbrot—a sourdough, coarse-grained bread
- Pumpernickel—very black; moist; with a smooth consistency
- Schwarzbrot (literally black bread)—made from a whole kernel grain; coarse
- süsse Brötchen—sweet rolls
- Vollkornbrot—a whole kernel grain again
- Weissbrot—white bread

If you are allergic to a specific grain, choose a flat bread (knäckebrot) that your diet allows; they are made with: *Weizen* (wheat), *Roggen* (rye), *Hafer* (oat), or *Reis* (rice).

■ **Please toast the bread.**
Bitte toasten Sie mein Brot.

■ **Please warm the _____.**
Bitten wärmen Sie der/die/das _____ auf.

- **Do you have bread or rolls baked without _____ or _____?**
  Haben Sie Brot oder Brötchen die ohne _____
  oder _____ gebacken worden sind?
  - fat—Fett
  - salt—Salz
  - sugar—Zucker
  - sweetening—süsse Zutaten

*Pfannkuchen* (pancakes) are much thinner than American-style pancakes. They usually contain a filling, like crepes, and are considered a luncheon dish rather than a breakfast food.

# Eggs—Eier

- fried—Spiegeleier
- hard-boiled—hart gekocht
- plain omelet—einfaches Omelet
- poached—verlorene Eier
- scrambled—Rührei
- soft-boiled—weich gekocht

# Dairy Products—
# Molkereiprodukte

There are three classifications of the fat content in dairy products: *vollfett* (full fat), *halbfett* (semifat, not exceeding 8 percent), and *mager* (almost fat-free). Also, look for the words *Magerstufe* and *fettarm,* which mean low-fat. Ask this question about dairy products:

- **Has it been refrigerated?**
  Ist es im Kühlschrank aufbewahrt worden?

### Butter—Butter
- sweet—süsse
- unsalted—ungesalzene

### Margarine—Margarine
- diet (low calorie)—Diät (wenig Kalorien)
- main ingredient should be unhardened (unsaturated) vegetable oil—sie sollte hauptsächlich aus ungehärtetem (ungesättigt) Pflanzenfett bestehen

## *Cheese—Käse*

Here are some questions you might want to ask about cheese:

- **Is it made with whole milk?**

  Ist der aus Vollmilch gemacht?

- **Is it made with skim milk?**

  Ist der aus Magermilch gemacht?

- **Is it made with part skim milk?**

  Ist der aus halbfetter Milch gemacht?

- **Has salt been added?**

  Ist Salz hinzugefügt worden?

- **What percentage of fat does it contain?**

  Wieviel Prozent Fett enhält es?

- **Please write it down. Thank you.**

  Bitte schreiben Sie es auf. Vielen Dank.

- **Do you have any _____ cheese?**

  Haben Sie Käse _____?
    - low-calorie—mit wenig Kalorien
    - low-fat—mit niedrigem Fettgehalt
    - low-salt—mit wenig Salz

- **Do you have any cottage cheese/pot cheese _____?**

  Haben Sie Quark _____?
    - plain/uncreamed—einfach/nicht cremig
    - salt-free—ohne Salz
    - sugar-free/unsweetened—ohne Zucker/ungesüsst

## *Cream—Sahne*
- nondairy creamer—künstliches Milchpulver
- sour—saure
- sweet—süsse

### *Milk—Milch*

- buttermilk—Buttermilch
- canned milk—Dosenmilch
  - condensed—kondensierte
  - evaporated skim—evaporierte Magermilch
  - evaporated whole—evaporierte Vollmilch
- fresh skim—frisch entrahmte
- fresh whole—frische Vollmilch
- homogenized—homogenisierte
- not homogenized—nicht homogenisierte
- pasteurized—pasteurisierte
- powdered skim milk/whole milk—Magermilchpulver/Vollmilchpulver

# Spreads

- honey—Honig
- jam—Konfitüre
- jelly—Gelee
- marmalade—Marmelade
- peanut butter—Erdnussbutter
  - chunky—mit Stückchen
  - freshly ground—frisch gemahlen
  - plain/smooth—einfach/ohne Stückchen
  - salt-free—ohne Salz
  - sugar-free (no sweetening)—ohne Zucker (ungesüsst)
  - without additives—ohne Zusatzstoffe
  - without hydrogenated oil—ohne hydrogenisiertes Öl

# Beverages — Getränke

- chocolate (cocoa)—Kakao
- coffee—Kaffee
- decaffeinated coffee—koffeinfreier Kaffee
- herb tea—Kräutertee
- tea—Tee

For an additional listing of beverages, see pages 131–132.

# Lunch and Dinner

## Main Courses

- meat—Fleisch
- poultry—Geflügel
- game—Wild
- fish—Fisch

Worried about preparation? Consult *Appendix 2: German Food Preparation.*
If you are curious about the meat in a dish on a menu, ask:

■ **What kind of meat is this?**
Was für Fleisch ist dies?

■ **Please show me on this list.**
Zeigen Sie es mir bitte auf dieser Liste.

■ **Do you have _____?**
Haben Sie _____?

■ **I would like _____.**
Ich möchte bitte _____.

■ **Please give me _____.**
Bitte geben Sie mir _____.

- chicken—Huhn, Hähnchen
- lamb—Hammelfleisch
- lean beef—mageres Rindfleisch
- pork—Schweinefleisch
- turkey—Putenfleisch
- veal—Kalbfleisch

Here are some cuts of meat, listed by category—beef, lamb, pork, poultry, veal, and variety meats.

# Cuts of Meat

## English—German
### Beef—*Rindfleisch*
- beefsteak—Rindersteak
- bottom round—unteres Rundstück
- chipped beef—schieres, geschnetzeltes Rindfleisch
- chuck—mageres Seitenstück
- flank steak—von der Flanke
- liver—Leber
- plate ribs—magere Rippen
- roast beef—Rinderbraten
- rump—vom Schwanzstück
- spare ribs—kurze Rippen
- steak—Steak
- tenderloin—Lendenstück
- top round—oberes Rundstück
- tripe—Flecke
- very lean baby beef—sehr mageres Kalbfleisch

### Lamb—*Hammel*
- leg—Keule
- loin chops—Lenden-Kottelets
- loin roast—Lendenbraten
- rib—Rippe
- shank—Beinstück
- shoulder—Schulter
- sirloin—Lendenstück

### Pork—*Schweinefleisch*
- center—Mittelstück
- cured ham—gesalzener Schinken

## German—English
### *Rindfleisch*—Beef
- Flecke—tripe
- kurze Rippen—spare ribs
- Leber—liver
- Lendenstück—tenderloin
- magere Rippen—plate ribs
- mageres Seitenstück—chuck
- oberes Rundstück—top round
- Rinderbraten—roast beef
- Rindersteak—beef steak
- schieres, geschnetzeltes Rindfleisch—chipped beef
- sehr mageres Kalbfleisch—very lean baby beef
- Steak—steak
- unteres Rundstück—bottom round
- vom Schwanzstück—rump
- von der Flanke—flank steak

### *Hammel*—Lamb
- Beinstück—shank
- Keule—leg
- Lendenbraten—loin roast
- Lenden-Kottelets—loin chops
- Lendenstück—sirloin
- Rippe—rib
- Schulter—shoulder

### *Schweinefleisch*—Pork
- alles Fett entfernt—well-trimmed
- Beinstück—leg

## English—German

- fresh ham—frischer Schinken
- leg—Beinstück
- pork chops—Schweinskoteletts
- rump—breites Schwanzstück
- shank—oberes Beinstück
- smoked ham (center slices)—geräucherter Schinken (Scheiben aus der Mitte)
- well-trimmed—alles Fett entfernt
- whole—im Stück

**Poultry—*Geflügel***
- chicken—Huhn
  - breast—Bruststück
  - leg—Keule
  - roast chicken—gebackenes Hähnchen
- Cornish hen—Hähnchen
- duck/duckling—Ente
- goose—Gans
- guinea hen—Perlhuhn
- partridge—Rebhuhn
- pheasant—Fasan
- pigeon—Taube
- quail—Wachtel
- turkey—Puten
  - breast—Bruststück
  - leg—Keule
  - roast turkey—gebackene Pute
- wild duck—Wildente
- wild squab—junge Wildtaube

## German—English

- breites Schwanzstück—rump
- frischer Schinken—fresh ham
- im Stück—whole
- geräucherter Schinken (Scheiben aus der Mitte)—smoked ham (center slices)
- gesalzener Schinken—cured ham
- Mittelstück—center
- oberes Beinstück—shank
- Schweinskoteletts—pork chops

***Geflügel*—Poultry**
- Ente—duck/duckling
- Fasan—pheasant
- Gans—goose
- Hähnchen—Cornish hen
- Huhn—chicken
  - Bruststück—breast
  - gebackenes Hähnchen—roast chicken
- Keule—leg
- junge Wildtaube—wild squab
- Perlhuhn—guinea hen
- Puten—turkey
  - Bruststück—breast
  - gebackene Pute—roast turkey
  - Keule—leg
- Rebhuhn—partridge
- Taube—pigeon
- Wachtel—quail
- Wildente—wild duck

*(continued on next page)*

German

Dining Out

# Cuts of Meat (continued)

*English—German*
**Veal—*Kalbfleisch***

- cutlets—Kottelets; boneless cutlets—Kalbsschnitzel
- leg—Beinstück
- loin—Lendenstück
- rib—Rippe
- shank—oberes Beinstück
- shoulder—Schulter
- slices (tenderloin)—Schnitzel

*German—English*
***Kalbfleisch*—Veal**

- Beinstück—leg
- Kalbsschnitzel—boneless cutlets
- Kottelets—cutlets
- Lendenstück—loin
- oberes Beinstück—shank
- Rippe—ribs
- Schnitzel—slices (tenderloin)
- Schulter—shoulder

## Other Meats and Variety Meats

- bacon—Speck
- blood sausage—Blutwurst
- brains—Gehirn
- chicken livers—Hühnerleber
- hare—Hase
- kidneys—Nieren
- minced meat—Gehacktes
- mutton—Hammel
- oxtail—Ochsenschwanz
- pig's feet—Schweinsfüsse
- sausages—Würste
- sweetbreads—Kalbsbröschen
- tongue—Zunge
- venison—Wildbret, Reh, Hirsch
- very lean ground meat (usually sirloin; served raw)—Tartar
- wild boar—Wildschwein
- wild rabbit—Wildkaninchen

- Blutwurst—blood sausage
- Gehacktes—minced meat
- Gehirn—brains
- Hammel—mutton
- Hase—hare
- Hirsch—venison
- Hühnerleber—chicken livers
- Kalbsbröschen—sweetbreads
- Nieren—kidneys
- Ochsenschwanz—oxtail
- Reh—venison
- Schweinsfüsse—pig's feet
- Speck—bacon
- Tartar—very lean ground meat (usually sirloin; served raw)
- Wildbret—venison
- Wildkaninchen—wild rabbit
- Wildschwein—wild boar
- Würste—sausages
- Zunge—tongue

German

Dining Out

# Fish — Fisch

- **What kind of fish is this?**
  Was für ein Fisch ist das?

- **Please show me on this list.**
  Zeigen Sie es mir bitte auf dieser Liste.

- **Is it fresh?**
  Ist er frisch?

- **Has it been frozen and thawed?**
  War er gefroren und ist aufgetaut worden?

- **Do you have _____?**
  Haben Sie _____?

- **I would like _____.**
  Ich möchte bitte _____.

- **Please give me _____.**
  Bitte geben Sie mir _____.

# Fresh and Saltwater Fish

*English — German*
- anchovies — Sardellen
- bass — Barsch
- bluefish — Goldmakrele
- bullhead — Kaulkopf
- carp — Karpfen
- clams — Venusmuscheln
- cod — Kabeljau
- conger eel — Seeaal
- crabs — Krebse
- crayfish — Flusskrebs
- eel — Aal
- flatfish — Plattfisch

*German — English*
- Aal — eel
- Austern — oysters
- Barsch — bass
- Brassen — sea bream
- Flunder — flounder
- Flussbarsch — perch
- Flusskrebs — crayfish
- Garnelen — shrimp
- geräucherter Lachs — smoked salmon
- Goldmakrele — bluefish
- Hecht — pike

*(continued on next page)*

German

Dining Out

# Fresh and Saltwater Fish
(continued)

## English—German

- flounder—Flunder
- haddock—Schellfisch
- halibut—Heilbutt
- herring—Hering
- lamprey—Neunauge
- lobster—Hummer
- mackerel—Makrele
- mussels—Muscheln
- octopus—Krake
- oysters—Austern
- perch—Flussbarsch
- pickerel—junger Hecht
- pike—Hecht
- pollock—Kalmück
- prawns—Krabben
- salmon—Lachs
  - smoked salmon—
    geräucherter Lachs
- sardines—Sardinen
- scallops—
  Jakobsmuscheln
- sea bream—Brassen
- shrimp—Garnelen
- smelt—Stint
- snapper—Schnapper
- sole—Seezunge
- sprats—Sprotten
- squid—Tintenfisch
  - baby squid—junger
    Tintenfisch
- sturgeon—Stör
- swordfish—Schwertfisch
- tuna—Thunfisch
- turbot—Steinbutt
- turtle—Schildkröte
- whitebait—kleiner
  Weissfisch
- whiting—Weissfisch

## German—English

- Heilbutt—halibut
- Hering—herring
- Hummer—lobster
- Jakobsmuscheln—
  scallops
- junger Hecht—pickerel
- junger Tintenfisch—
  baby squid
- Kabeljau—cod
- Kalmück—pollock
- Karpfen—carp
- Kaulkopf—bullhead
- kleiner Weissfisch—
  whitebait
- Krabben—prawns
- Krake—octopus
- Krebse—crabs
- Lachs—salmon
- Makrele—mackerel
- Muscheln—mussels
- Neunauge—lamprey
- Plattfisch—flatfish
- Sardellen—anchovies
- Sardinen—sardines
- Schellfisch—haddock
- Schildkröte—turtle
- Schnapper—snapper
- Schwertfisch—swordfish
- Seeaal—conger eel
- Seezunge—sole
- Sprotten—sprats
- Steinbutt—turbot
- Stint—smelt
- Stör—sturgeon
- Thunfisch—tuna
- Tintenfisch—squid
- Venusmuscheln—clams
- Weissfisch—whiting

German

Dining Out

# Vegetables – Gemüse

- **Do you have _____?**
  Haben Sie _____?

- **I would like _____.**
  Ich möchte bitte _____.

- **Please give me _____.**
  Bitte geben Sie mir _____.

# Vegetables

## English – German

- artichokes – Artischocken
- asparagus – Spargel
- beets – rote Bete
- brussels sprouts – Rosenkohl
- cabbage – Kohl
  - red cabbage – Rotkohl
- capers – Kapern
- carrots – Karotten
- cauliflower – Blumenkohl
- celery – Selerie
- chick-peas – Kichererbsen
- chicory – Zichorie
- chili – Chili
- chives – Schnittlauch
- corn (on the cob) – Maiskolben
- cucumber – Gurken
- eggplant – Aubergine
- endive – Endivien
- garlic – Knoblauch
- gherkins – kleine Gurken
- green beans – grüne Bohnen

## German – English

- Artischocken – artichokes
- Aubergine – eggplant
- Blumenkohl – cauliflower
- Chili – chili
- Endivien – endive
- Erbsen – peas
- grüne Bohnen – green beans
- Gurken – cucumber
- junge Paprikaschoten – sweet peppers
- Kapern – capers
- Karotten – carrots
- Kartoffeln – potatoes
- Kichererbsen – chick-peas
- kleine Gurken – gherkins
- Knoblauch – garlic
- Kohl – cabbage
- Linsen – lentils
- Maiskolben – corn (on the cob)
- Markkürbis – zucchini
- Paprikaschoten – peppers
- Pastinaken – parsnips
- Petersilie – parsley

*(continued on next page)*

# Vegetables (continued)

*English—German*
- leeks—Porree
- lentils—Linsen
- lettuce—Salat
- mushrooms—Pilze
- onions—Zwiebeln
- parsley—Petersilie
- parsnips—Pastinaken
- peas—Erbsen
- peppers—Paprikaschoten
- potatoes—Kartoffeln
- radishes—Radieschen
- red cabbage—Rotkohl
- rice—Reis
- saffron—Safran
- spinach—Spinat
- sweet peppers—junge Paprikaschoten
- sweet potatoes—Süsskartoffeln
- tomatoes—Tomaten
- truffles—Trüffeln
- yams—James, Süsskartoffelwurzeln
- zucchini—Markkürbis, Zuckini

*German—English*
- Pilze—mushrooms
- Porree—leeks
- Radieschen—radishes
- Reis—rice
- Rosenkohl—brussels sprouts
- rote Bete—beets
- Rotkohl—red cabbage
- Safran—saffron
- Salat—salad
- Schnittlauch—chives
- Selerie—celery
- Spargel—asparagus
- Spinat—spinach
- Süsskartoffeln—sweet potatoes
- Süsskartoffelwurzeln—yams
- Tomaten—tomatoes
- Trüffeln—truffles
- Zichorie—chicory
- Zuckini—zucchini
- Zwiebeln—onions

# Pasta—Teigwaren

- **Please cook it in unsalted water.**
  Bitte kochen Sie es in ungesalzenem Wasser.

- **Was this cooked in salted water?**
  Ist dies in Salzwasser gekocht worden?

- **Please ask the chef to check the label on the container. Does it contain any _____?**
  Würden Sie den Koch bitten, die Aufschrift auf der Packung zu lesen? Enthält es irgendeine Art von _____?
  - egg—Ei
  - salt—Salz
  - sugar—Zucker
  - sweetening—Süssstoffen

### Pasta Products
- farina dumplings—Griessknödel
- macaroni—Makaroni
- noodles—Nudeln
- small (wheat) dumplings—Spätzle
- spaghetti—Spagetti
- spinach noodles—grüne Nudeln
- vermicelli—Vermicelli
- white flour—weisses Mehl
- whole wheat—Vollweizenmehl

# Soft Drinks – Erfrischungsgetränke

- **Do you have _____?**
  Haben Sie _____?

- **I would like _____.**
  Ich möchte bitte _____.

- **Please give me _____.**
  Bitte geben Sie mir _____.

German

Dining Out

131

- **a glass/bottle/can of** _____.
  ein Glas/eine Flasche/eine Dose _____.

  • with (a lot of) ice—mit (viel) Eis
- bouillon—Bouillon
- Coke—Cola
- fruit juice—Fruchtsaft
- iced coffee—Eiskaffee
- lemonade—Limonade
- lemon soda—Zitronenlimonade
- milk shake—Milchshake
- milk soda—Milchsoda
- mineral water—Mineralwasser
- orange soda—Orangensprudel
- vegetable juice—Gemüsesaft
- Viennese iced coffee—Wiener Eis–Kaffee

For a larger selection of beverages, see pages 115 and 122.

# Alcoholic Drinks — alkoholische Getränke

- **Do you have** _____?
  Haben Sie _____?

- **I would like** _____.
  Ich möchte bitte _____.

- **Please give me** _____.
  Bitte geben Sie mir _____.

- a glass—ein Glas
- a half-bottle—halbe Flasche
- a bottle—eine Flasche
- one liter—einen Liter
- a beer—ein Bier
- red wine—Rotwein
- white wine—Weisswein
- sweet wine—Süsswein
- very dry wine—einen sehr trockenen Wein

# Part 3

## The Low-Sodium (Low-Salt) Diet

The following list of "not permitted" items may vary from the list of foods your physician has instructed you to avoid. To make the list easier for others to read, cross out the items that do not apply to you and write in, PRINTING LEGIBLY, any other things you must avoid. Select them from the food lists on pages 114–132.

To make sure your food and drinks are prepared properly, consult *Appendix 2: German Food Preparation.* Use it together with other appropriate pages when ordering meals.

Keep in mind that there are hidden sources of sodium in most cooking. Baked goods may be made with baking soda (sodium bicarbonate) or baking powder rather than yeast, and you know, of course, that baking powder contains sodium. Ask:

■ **Is this made with baking powder/baking soda or yeast?**

Ist dies mit *Backpulver/Backsoda/Natron* oder Hefe zubereitet?

Beware also that antacids, like Alka Seltzer, and other indigestion aids may contain sodium bicarbonate or other sodium compounds. Before you go abroad, ask your physician to suggest a low-sodium antacid to take with you. If you must buy an antacid in Germany, check the labels for any of these terms: *Sodium Bicarbonat, Natron, Natrium,* or the international symbol *Na.* If you are shopping for food, your checklist for sodium compounds should also include *doppeltkohlensaures Natron* which is used for baking soda on some product labels.

Finally, check the labels on bottled mineral waters for sodium content. The table on page 27 can serve as a guideline.

So far all you've read is *avoid, not permitted, beware,* and you're wondering what you can eat or drink in Germany and still stick to your diet. Your diet scenario will sound pretty negative too, but don't let that frighten you. Take a look at the extensive food lists in *Part 2* of this section, pages 114–132. If you can't order from the menu the waiter gives you, ask for items selected from the food lists. Combine your selections with information from *Appendix 2: German Food Preparation* and the diet scenario that follows to produce a satisfying meal, one custom-made to your specifications.

If you are planning to stay at a hotel more than a few days and take most of your meals there, you might want to ask the maitre d' to provide salt-free bread for you. Explain:

■ **I am on a salt-free diet and cannot eat bread or baked goods that contain salt or baking powder.**

Ich halte mich an eine salzfreie Diät und darf kein Brot oder andere Backwaren mit Salz oder Backpulver essen.

■ **I would appreciate it very much if you could get salt-free bread for my meals.**

Ich wäre Ihnen sehr dankbar, wenn Sie mir salzfreies Brot für meine Mahlzeiten geben könnten.

Remember: bread is not normally served with meals, and you will have to ask for it. Of course, you will be charged extra too.

# Foods Not Permitted – Verbotenes Essen

- anchovies—Sardellen
- anything baked with baking powder or baking soda— alles Gebackene mit Backpulver oder Backsoda
- bacon drippings— Schweinefett
- baking soda—Backsoda (Natron)
- bouillon—Bouillon
- broth—Fleischbrühe
- canned fish—Fisch in Dosen
- canned meat—Dosenfleisch
- canned tomatoes—Tomaten in Dosen
- canned vegetables— Dosengemüse
- capers—Kapern
- catsup—Katchup
- celery salt—Selleriesalz
- cheese—Käse
- chili powder—Chili–Puder

- chili sauce—Chili-Sauce
- chive—Schnittlauch
- condensed milk—Kondensmilch
- cured meats—geräuchertes Fleisch
- garlic salt—Knoblauchsalz
- gravy—Sosse
- horseradish—Meerrettich
- instant or frozen potatoes—getrocknete oder gefrorene Kartoffeln (Schnellkartoffeln)
- margarine—Margarine
- mayonnaise—Mayonnaise
- meat sauce—Fleischsosse
- milk—Milch
- monosodium glutamate (MSG)—Monosodium Glutamat
- mustard—Senf
- relish—gewürzte Beilagen
- salt—Salz
- salted butter—gesalzene Butter
- salted salad dressing—Salatsauce mit Salz
- sausage—Wurst
- seasoned salt—Gewürzsalz
- sodium preservatives—Sodium (Natrium) Frischhaltemittel
- soy sauce—Soja-Sauce
- tomato puree—Tomatenpaste
- tomato sauce—Tomatensauce

# The Low-Sodium (Low-Salt) Scenario

- **salt-free diet**
  Salzfreie Diät

If you can't pronounce the German, point to appropriate phrases. For some sample replies to your questions, turn to *Appendix 2: German Food Preparation* and show it to your respondent.

- **I have a reservation. My name is _____.**
  Ich habe eine Vorbestellung. Mein Name ist _____.

- **Please tell the manager I am here.**
  Bitte sagen Sie dem Manager, dass ich hier bin.

- **The manager knows about the special service I need because of a medical problem.**
  Der Manager weiss von der benötigten Extrabehandlung wegen meines Gesundheitszustandes.

135

- **Does anyone here speak English?**
Spricht hier jemand Englisch?

- **I/she/he must follow a special diet.**
Ich/sie/er muss eine besondere Diät einhalten.

- **All my food and drink must be completely salt-free.**
Meine Speisen und Getränke müssen vollkommen salzfrei sein.

- **Everything must be prepared without the items on this list.**
Alles muss ohne die Zutaten auf dieser Liste zubereitet werden.

- **A mistake can cause serious illness.**
Ein Versehen kann zu einer ernsthaften Krankheit bei mir führen.

- **Does this dish contain any salt?**
Enthält dieses Essen Salz?

- **Does this dish contain anything on this list?**
Enthält dieses Essen irgendwelche Zutaten von der Liste?

- **Can you prepare this dish without salt?**
Könnten Sie dieses Gericht ohne Salz zubereiten?

- **Can you prepare this dish without any of the items on this list?**
Könnten Sie dieses Gericht ohne die Zutaten auf dieser Liste zubereiten?

- **Show me on the menu which dishes you can prepare without salt.**
Bitte zeigen Sie mir, welche Gerichte auf der Speisekarte ohne Salz zubereitet werden können.

- **Show me on the menu which dishes you can prepare without any of the items on this list?**
  Bitte zeigen Sie mir, welche Gerichte auf der Speisekarte ohne die Zutaten auf dieser Liste zubereitet werden können.

- **Which dishes on the menu are salt-free?**
  Welche Gerichte auf der Speisekarte sind salzfrei?

- **Are there any dishes on the menu that do not contain ingredients forbidden to me?**
  Gibt es Gerichte auf der Speisekarte, die keine der mir verbotenen Zutaten enthalten?

- **Are the tomatoes in this dish fresh, frozen or canned? (Waiter, please point to the right word.)**
  Sind die Tomaten in diesem Gericht frisch, gefroren oder aus der Dose? (Herr Ober, bitte zeigen Sie auf das passende Wort.)

- **Is the pasta cooked in salted water?**
  Sind die Nudeln in Salzwasser gekocht?

- **Can you prepare a serving of pasta for me, cooked in unsalted water?**
  Könnten Sie eine Portion Nudeln für mich in ungesalzenem Wasser kochen?

- **Are the potatoes/vegetables cooked in salted water?**
  Sind ist die Kartoffeln/das Gemüse in Salzwasser gekocht?

- **Can you prepare potatoes/vegetables for me in unsalted water?**
  Könnten Sie Kartoffeln/Gemüse für mich in ungesalzenem Wasser kochen?

Low-Sodium Diet

137

- **If you are not sure, please tell me/ask the chef/the maitre d'.**
Wenn Sie nicht ganz sicher sind, sagen Sie es mir bitte/fragen Sie bitte den Koch/Oberkellner.

- **I would like to speak to the chef/the maitre d'.**
Ich möchte gern mit dem Koch/dem Oberkellner sprechen.

- **Can you prepare something simple and salt-free for me in your kitchen? For example, plain baked or broiled fish; steak; baked, boiled, or mashed potatoes; fresh, cooked, unsalted vegetables? Potatoes and vegetables must not be cooked in salted water.**
Könnten Sie etwas Einfaches, Salzfreies für mich zubereiten? Zum Beispiel, ungesalzenen, gebak-kenen oder auf dem Rost gebratenen Fisch, Steak; gebackene oder gekochte Kartoffeln, Stampfkar-toffeln; frisches, ungesalzenes Gemüse? Die Kartoffeln und das Gemüse müssen in ungesalzenem Wasser gekocht werden.

- **Do you have a microwave oven/a pressure cooker?**
Haben Sie einen Microwellen-Ofen/einen Schnell-kocher?

(If the answer is *yes,* then ask:)

- **Can you prepare a portion of _____, plain/without seasoning/ gravy/sauce/salt?**
Könnten Sie eine Einzelportion von _____ ohne jegliche Gewürze/Sosse/Sauce/Salz zubereiten?

- **A mistake has been made. This is not what I ordered.**
Hier liegt ein Versehen vor. Dies habe ich nicht bestellt.

# The Diabetic Diet

Your physician has outlined your diet and probably shown you how to select balanced meals using a system of food exchanges. The phrases in this section will help you identify dishes on a menu that contain added sweetening. If you must also observe a low-fat, low-cholesterol diet, refer to the scenario for that diet on page 143.

**Caution:** If you must take an antacid, be sure to read the information on page 15 about the sugar content of many popular antacids.

To make sure your food and drinks are properly prepared, consult *Appendix 2: German Food Preparation*. Use it together with other appropriate pages when ordering meals.

Check the "not permitted" list. To make it easier for others to read, cross out the items that do not apply to you, and add, PRINTING LEGIBLY, other things you cannot have. Select them from the food lists on pages 114–132.

---

## Foods Not Permitted – Verbotenes Essen

- butter—Butter
- condensed milk—Kondensmilch
- corn sweetener—Maiszucker
- corn syrup—Maissyrup
- dextrose—Dextrose
- fats—Fette
- fructose—Fruchtzucker
- honey—Honig
- jam—Konfitüre
- jelly—Gelee
- lard—Talg
- maltose—Malzzucker
- margarine—Margarine
- marmalade—Marmelade
- molasses—Melasse
- oils—Öle
- rice syrup—Reissyrup
- shortening—Backfett
- sugar—Zucker
- sugar-beet syrup—Rübenzucker
- syrup—Syrup

---

## The Diabetic Scenario

If you cannot pronounce the German, point to the appropriate phrases. For some sample replies to your questions, turn to *Appendix 2: German Food Preparation* and show it to your respondent.

■ **I have a reservation. My name is _____.**
Ich habe eine Vorbestellung. Mein Name ist _____.

■ **Please tell the manager I am here.**
Bitte sagen Sie dem Manager, dass ich hier bin.

■ **The manager knows about the special service I need because of a medical problem.**
Der Manager weiss von der benötigten Extra-behandlung wegen meines Gesundheitszustandes.

■ **Does anyone here speak English?**
Spricht hier jemand Englisch?

■ **I/she/he must follow a special diet because of diabetes.**
Ich/sie/er muss mich/sich wegen Zuckerkrankheit eine spezielle Diät einhalten.

■ **All my food and drink must be free of added sugar or sweetening.**
Mein Essen und meine Getränke dürfen keinen Extra-Zucker enthalten.

■ **Everything must be prepared without the ingredients on this list.**
Alles muss ohne die Zutaten auf dieser Liste zubereitet werden.

■ **A mistake can cause serious illness.**
Ein Versehen kann eine ernsthafte Krankheit herbei-führen.

- **Does this dish/beverage/juice contain any of the sweeteners on the list?**

  Enthält dieses Essen/Getränk/dieser Saft irgend-welche süssen Zutaten von der Liste?

- **Can you prepare this dish/juice/beverage without sweetening?**

  Könnten Sie dieses Essen/diesen Saft/dieses Getränk ohne süsse Zutaten zubereiten?

- **Are the fruits/vegetables in this dish fresh/canned/frozen?**

  Sind diese Früchte/dieses Gemüse frisch/aus der Dose/gefroren?

- **If it is canned or frozen in syrup, please drain all the liquid.**

  Falls die Dose oder die Gefrierpackung Syrup enthält, giessen Sie bitte den Syrup aus.

- **Do you have any artificial sweetener?**

  Haben Sie künstliche Süssstoffe?

- **If you are not sure, please tell me/ask the chef/the maitre d'.**

  Falls Sie nicht sicher sind, Sagen Sie es mir bitte/fragen Sie den Koch/den Oberkellner.

- **Do you have a microwave oven/a pressure cooker?**

  Haben Sie einen Microwellen-Ofen/einen Schnell-kocher?

  (If the answer is *yes*, then ask:)

- **Can you prepare a portion of _____, plain/without seasoning/gravy/sauce/sugar/sweetening?**

  Könnten Sie eine Einzelportion von _____ ohne jegliche Gewürze / Sosse / Sauce / Zucker / andere Süssstoffe zubereiten?

- **A mistake has been made. This is not what I ordered.**
  Es handelt sich hier um ein Versehen. Das habe ich nicht bestellt.

- **I would like to speak to the chef/the maitre d'.**
  Ich möchte mit dem Koch/dem Oberkellner sprechen.

# The Low-Fat and Low-Cholesterol Diet

The following list of "not-permitted" items may vary from the foods your physician has instructed you to avoid. To make the list easier for others to read, cross out the items that do not apply to you and add, PRINTING LEGIBLY, other things you must avoid. Select them from the food lists on pages 114–132.

To make sure your food and drinks are prepared properly, consult *Appendix 2: German Food Preparation.* Use it together with other appropriate pages when ordering meals.

German cuisine can be rough on a low-fat, low-cholesterol diet, but if you stick to simple dishes that can be made to order, you will be able to maintain your diet. Stay away from stews and casseroles; they are apt to be quite fatty. When ordering meat, have the fat trimmed before it's broiled or baked. And remember, the necessary phrases are in your scenario and the preparation appendix.

## Foods Not Permitted – Verbotenes Essen

- all animal fats—alle Tierfette
- all fats—alle Fette
- all oils—alle Öle
- avocado—Avocado
- bacon fat—Schmalz
- butter—Butter
- canned meat/fish— Dosenfleisch/Fisch
- cheese sauces—Käse- Saucen

- cheese/yogurt made with whole or part skim milk— Voll oder Magermilch Käse/Yoghurt
- chocolate—Schokolade
- cocoa—Kakao
- coconut—Kokosnuss
- coconut oil—Kokosnussöl
- cream—Sahne
- eggs—Eier
- egg yolk—Eigelb
- fried foods—Gebratenes
- gravy—Bratensosse
- ground meat—Hackfleisch
- heart—Herz
- hydrogenated oil—hydrogeniertes Öl
- kidney—Nieren
- lard—Talg
- liver—Leber
- margarine—Margarine
- mayonnaise—Mayonnaise
- nuts—Nüsse
- olive oil—Olivenöl
- palm kernel oil—Palmenkernöl
- palm oil—Palmöl
- part skim milk—Magermilch
- peanut oil—Erdnussöl
- (oil) salad dressing—(Öl) Salatsaucen
- sausage—Wurst
- shortening—Bratfett
- shrimp—Krabben
- sour cream—Saure Sahne
- sweetbreads—Gehirn
- whole milk—Vollmilch

# The Low-Fat and Low-Cholesterol Scenario

If you can't pronounce the German, point to the appropriate phrases. For some sample replies to your questions, turn to *Appendix 2: German Food Preparation* and show it to your respondent.

■ **I have a reservation. My name is _____.**

Ich habe eine Vorbestellung. Mein Name ist _____.

■ **Please tell the manager I am here.**

Bitte sagen Sie dem Manager, dass ich hier bin.

■ **The manager knows about the special service I need because of a medical problem.**

Der Manager weiss von der benötigten Extrabehandlung wegen meines Gesundheitszustandes.

- **Does anyone here speak English?**
  Spricht hier jemand Englisch?

- **I/she/he must follow a special diet because of a serious medical problem.**
  Ich/sie/er muss eine spezielle Diät einhalten, wegen eines Gesundheitsproblems.

- **All food and drink must be fat-free.**
  Mein Essen und meine Getränke dürfen kein Fett enthalten.

- **Everything must be prepared without the ingredients on this list.**
  Alles muss ohne die Zutaten auf der Lister zubereitet werden.

- **Nothing can be fried.**
  Nichts darf gebraten werden.

- **All visible fat must be trimmed before cooking.**
  Das ganze Fett muss abgeschnitten werden vor dem Kochen.

- **A mistake can cause serious illness.**
  Ein Versehen kann eine ernsthafte Krankheit herbeiführen.

- **Does this dish contain any _____?**
  Enthält dieses Gericht _____?

- **Can you prepare this dish without _____?**
  Könnten Sie dieses Gericht ohne _____ zubereiten?

- **Can you prepare this dish with _____ instead of _____?**
  Könnten Sie dieses Gericht mit _____ anstatt _____ zubereiten?

144

- **Does this dish contain anything on this list?**
Enthält dieses Gericht etwas von der Liste?

- **Can you prepare this dish without any of the items on this list?**
Könnten Sie dieses Gericht ohne irgendwelche Zutaten von der Liste zubereiten?

- **Are there any dishes on your menu that do not contain ingredients forbidden to me?**
Gibt es Gerichte auf ihrer Speisekarte, die keine der mir verbotenen Zutaten enthalten?

- **Can you fry/prepare this dish with any of these oils: safflower/sunflower/corn/soy/cottonseed/peanut?**
Könnten Sie dieses Gericht braten/zubereiten/mit irgendeinem dieser Öle: Safran/Sonnenblumen/Mais/Soyabohnen/Erdnuss?

- **Please serve this plain, without any sauce/gravy.**
Bitte servieren Sie dies einfach, ohne Sauce/Bratensosse.

- **If you are not sure, please tell me/ask the chef/the maitre d'.**
Falls Sie nicht sicher sind, sagen Sie es mir bitte/fragen Sie den Koch/den Oberkellner.

- **I would like to speak to the chef/the maitre d'.**
Ich möchte gerne mit dem Koch/dem Oberkellner sprechen.

- **Do you have a microwave oven/a pressure cooker?**
Haben Sie einen Microwellen-Ofen/einen Schnellkocher?

(If the answer is *yes*, then ask:)

German

Low-Fat/Low-Cholesterol Diet

- **Can you prepare a single portion of _____, plain/without seasoning/gravy/sauce/butter/oil/fats?**
  Könnten Sie eine Einzelportion von _____ ohne jegliche Gewürze/Braten Sosse/Sauce/Butter/Öl/Fett zubereiten?

- **A mistake has been made. This is not what I ordered.**
  Hier liegt ein Versehen vor. Ich habe das nicht bestellt.

## The Ulcer, Bland, Soft, and Low-Residue Diet

The items on the following list may vary from the foods your physician has instructed you to avoid. To make the list easier for others to read, cross out the items that do not apply to you and add, PRINTING LEGIBLY, the things you cannot have. Select them from the food lists on pages 114–132.

To make sure your food and drinks are prepared properly, consult *Appendix 2: German Food Preparation*. Use it together with other appropriate pages when ordering meals.

## Foods Not Permitted – Verbotenes Essen

- bran—Kleie
- brown/wild rice—brauner/ wilder Reis
- catsup—Katchup
- chili—Chili
- clams—Venusmuscheln
- coarse bread—grobes Brot
- coarse cereals—grobe Getreidespeisen
- coconut—Kokosnuss
- corn—Mais

- dried fruits—getrocknete Früchte
- dried legumes—getrocknete Hülsenfrüchte
- fat—Fett
- foods prepared with wine or liqueurs—Speisen mit Wein oder anderen alkoholischen Getränken zubereitet
- fried foods—gebratene Speisen

- garlic—Knoblauch
- gravy—Sosse
- herbs—Gewürz-Kräuter
- horseradish—Meerrettich
- lard—Talg
- meat broth—Fleischbrühe
- mustard—Senf
- nuts/seeds—Nüsse/Kerne
- olives—Oliven
- onions—Zwiebeln
- oysters—Austern
- paprika—Paprika
- peas—Erbsen
- pepper—Pfeffer
- pickled meat/fish—Fleisch/ Fisch, eingelegt
- pork—Schweinefleisch
- raisins—Rosinen
- relish—pikante Beigaben
- salt—Salz
- sauce—Sauce
- seasoning—Würze
- sharp (strong) cheese— scharfer Käse
- spices—Gewürze
- vinegar—Essig

# The Ulcer, Bland, Soft, and Low-Residue Scenario

If you cannot pronounce the German, point to appropriate phrases. For some sample replies to your questions, turn to *Appendix 2: German Food Preparation* and show it to your respondent.

■ **I have a reservation. My name is _____.**

Ich habe eine Vorbestellung. Mein Name ist _____.

■ **Please tell the manager I am here.**

Bitte sagen Sie dem Manager, dass ich hier bin.

■ **The manager knows about the special service I need because of a medical problem.**

Der Manager weiss von der benötigten Extrabehandlung wegen meines Gesundheitszustandes.

■ **Does anyone here speak English?**

Spricht hier jemand Englisch?

■ **I/she/he must follow a special diet for a stomach problem.**
Ich/sie/er muss wegen eines Magenproblems eine besondere Diät einhalten.

■ **Everything must be prepared without spices/seasoning.**
Alle Speisen müssen ohne Gewürze zubereitet werden.

■ **Nothing can be fried. Food must be baked/broiled/stewed/ poached.***
Nichts darf gebraten werden. Das Essen muss gebacken/auf dem Rost geschmort/gedämpft/ gesiedet werden.

■ **A mistake can cause serious illness.**
Ein Versehen kann eine ernsthafte Krankheit herbeiführen.

■ **Please bake/broil/stew/poach* this dish.**
Bitte backen/schmoren/dämpfen/sieden Sie diese Speise.

■ **Can you bake/broil/stew/poach* this dish?**
Könnten Sie diese Speise backen/schmoren/ dämpfen/sieden?

■ **Everything must be prepared without the ingredients on this list. Please read it. Thank you.**
Alles muss ohne die Zutaten auf dieser Liste zubereitet werden. Bitte lesen Sie es. Vielen Dank.

■ **Does this dish contain any _____?**
Enthält diese Speise _____?

*gesiedet—poached (fish); verlorene Eier—poached eggs

■ **Can you prepare this dish without _____?**
Könnten Sie diese Speise ohne _____ zubereiten?

■ **Can you prepare this dish with _____ instead of _____?**
Könnten Sie diese Speise mit _____ anstatt _____ zubereiten?

■ **If you are not sure, please tell me/ask the chef/the maitre d'.**
Wenn Sie nicht ganz sicher sind, sagen Sie es mir bitte/fragen Sie bitte den Koch/den Oberkellner.

■ **Can you prepare something bland and simple like a platter of plain baked fish, baked potato or plain boiled potatoes, tender carrots or spinach or green beans or mushrooms?**
Könnten Sie etwas Einfaches,Ungewürztes zubereiten, wie einfachen, gebackenen Fisch, eine gebackene Kartoffel oder gekochte Kartoffeln, weiche Karotten oder zarten Spinat oder grüne Bohnen oder Pilze ohne Zutaten?

■ **Do you have a microwave oven/pressure cooker?**
Haben Sie einen Microwellen-Ofen/einen Schnellkocher?

(If the answer is *yes*, then ask:)

■ **Can you prepare a portion of _____, plain/without seasoning/gravy/sauce?**
Könnten Sie eine einfache Einzelportion von _____ ohne jegliche Gewürze/Sosse/Sauce zubereiten?

■ **A mistake has been made. This is not what I ordered.**
Hier liegt ein Versehen vor. Dies habe ich nicht bestellt.

■ **I would like to speak with the chef/the maitre d'.**
Ich möchte gern mit dem Koch/dem Oberkellner sprechen.

German

Ulcer, Low-Residue Diet

149

# Design Your Own Scenario for a Custom-made Diet

If, for health, personal, or religious reasons, you require a special diet that does not appear in this repertoire, you can produce your own script. We've made it easy for you by supplying the phrases on the following pages. To fill in the blanks in the phrases you plan to use, do the following:

**1.** On a separate sheet of paper, prepare a list of foods you cannot eat.

**2.** Translate them into German by consulting the "not permitted" lists of the other diets and the food lists on pages 114–132; you may also find the supplementary lists at the end of this chapter useful.

**3.** Copy the list into this book, PRINTING LEGIBLY, in the blank spaces provided under the heading, "not permitted." PRINT it in German *and* English.

**4.** PRINT the German words, where applicable, in the blanks we've provided.

**5.** Don't forget to use *Appendix 2: German Food Preparation* to explain how you want your food prepared.

| **Foods Not Permitted** | **Verbotenes Essen** |
|---|---|
| | |
| | |
| | |
| | |
| | |
| | |
| | |
| | |
| | |
| | |
| | |
| | |
| | |
| | |
| | |

# The Custom-made Scenario

If you can't pronounce the German, point to appropriate phrases. For some sample replies to your questions, turn to *Appendix 2: German Food Preparation* and show it to your respondent.

■ **I have a reservation. My name is _____.**
Ich habe eine Vorbestellung. Mein Name ist _____.

■ **Please tell the manager I am here.**
Bitte sagen Sie dem Manager, dass ich hier bin.

■ **The manager knows about the special service I need because of a medical problem.**
Der Manager weiss von der benötigten Extrabehandlung wegen meines Gesundheitszustandes.

■ **The manager knows about the special diet I need.**
Der Manager weiss von der speziellen Diät, die ich einhalte.

■ **Does anyone here speak English?**
Spricht hier jemand Englisch?

■ **I/she/he must follow a special diet.**
Ich/sie/er muss eine spezielle Diät einhalten.

■ **All my food and drink must be prepared without _____.**
Mein ganzes Essen und alle meine Getränke müssen ohne _____ zubereitet werden.

■ **Everything must be prepared without the items on this list.**
Alles muss ohne die Zutaten von der Liste zubereitet werden.

- **A mistake can cause serious illness.**

Ein Versehen kann eine ernsthafte Krankheit herbeiführen.

- **Does this dish contain any _____?**

Enthält dieses Gericht _____?

- **Does this dish contain anything on this list?**

Enthält dieses Gericht etwas von dieser Liste?

- **Can you prepare this dish without _____?**

Könnten Sie dieses Gericht ohne _____ zubereiten?

- **Show me on the menu which dishes you can prepare without _____.**

Zeigen Sie mir bitte auf der Speisekarte welche Gerichte Sie ohne _____ zubereiten können.

- **Show me on the menu which dishes you can prepare without any of the items on this list.**

Zeigen Sie mir auf der Speisekarte welche Gerichte Sie ohne die Zutaten auf der Liste zubereiten können.

- **Are there any dishes on the menu that do not contain ingredients forbidden to me?**

Gibt es Gerichte auf ihrer Speisekarte, die keine der mir verbotenen Zutaten enthalten?

- **If you are not sure, please tell me/ask the chef/the maitre d'.**

Falls Sie nicht sicher sind, sagen Sie es mir bitte/ fragen Sie den Koch/den Oberkellner.

- **I would like to speak to the chef/the maitre d'.**

Ich möchte mit dem Koch/dem Oberkellner sprechen.

- **Can you prepare something simple for me in your kitchen that is appropriate for my diet? For example: _____.**
  Könnten Sie etwas Einfaches für mich kochen, das in meine Diät passt? Zum Beispiel: _____.

- **Do you have a microwave oven/a pressure cooker?**
  Haben Sie einen Microwellen-Ofen/einen Schnellkocher?

  (If the answer is *yes*, then ask:)

- **Can you prepare a portion of _____ without _____?**
  Könnten Sie eine einfache Einzelportion von _____ ohne _____ zubereiten?

- **A mistake has been made. This is not what I ordered.**
  Ein Versehen liegt hier vor. Das habe ich nicht bestellt.

To compose a list of forbidden items consult the food lists on pages 114–132, the collection of no-nos for the other scenarios, and this sampling of foods that may cause reactions in some allergenic and otherwise sensitive individuals.

# Possible Forbidden Items — Verbotenes Essen

- barley—Gerste
- barley cereal—Gerste-oder Graupennährmittel
- barley flour—Gerstenmehl
- barley soup—Gerstensuppe-oder Graupensuppe
- beef—Rindfleisch
- beets—Rüben, Bete
- bran—Kleie
- buckwheat—Buchweizen
- buckwheat cereal—Buchweizennährmittel
- buckwheat flour—Buchweizenmehl
- buckwheat stuffing—Füllung mit Buchweizen
- chocolate—Schokolade
- cinnamon—Zimt
- citrus fruits—Zitrusfrüchte
- coconut—Kokosnuss

*(continued on next page)*

# Possible Forbidden Items—
# Verbotenes Essen (continued)

- coffee—Kaffee
- cola—Cola
- corn—Mais
- corn products—Mais-Produkte
- dates—Datteln
- eggs—Eier
- figs—Feigen
- fish—Fisch
- flax seeds—Flachssamen
- legumes—Hülsenfrüchte
- lettuce—Salat
- malt—Malz
- malt coloring—Malz als Farbstoff
- malt flavoring—Malz als Geschmackstoff
- milk—Milch
- nuts—Nüsse
- oat flour—Hafermehl
- oatmeal bread—Brot mit Hafer (flocken)
- oatmeal cereal—Nährmittel mit Haferflocken
- oatmeal stuffing—Füllung mit Haferflocken
- oats—Hafer
- peanuts—Erdnüsse

- pork—Schweinefleisch
- potato—Kartoffeln
- rice—Reis
- ripe beans—reife Bohnen
- rye—Roggen
- rye bread—Roggenbrot
- rye bread crumbs—Roggenbrotkrümel
- rye cereal—Roggennährmittel
- rye flour—Roggenmehl
- shellfish—Schalentiere
- soybeans—Soja-Bohnen
- string beans—grüne Bohnen
- tomato—Tomaten
- wheat—Weizen
- wheat bread—Weizenbrot
- wheat cereal—Weizennährmittel
- wheat crumbs—Weizenkrümel
- wheat flour—Weizenmehl
- wheat germ—Weizenkeime
- wheat germ oil—Weizenkeimöl
- wheat stuffing—Füllung mit Weizen
- yeast—Hefe

# Medical Aid

Read these pages now. They will make things easier for you later.

In an acute emergency ask a German-speaking person to telephone for help for you. You will find the phrase for such a request under *Emergencies* on page 156. Memorize it now.

## U.S. Embassy and Consular Assistance in Germany

If you are visiting Bonn, you can obtain a list of qualified English-speaking physicians from the American Embassy. It's a good thing to keep handy. Why wait for an emergency? Get your umbrella before it rains! Drop in for your list at the:

**Embassy of the United States** — Bonn, Delchmann-saue. Telephone: (0228) 339-3390.

Consular services are available in other German cities, too:

**Berlin** — Clayallee 170. Telephone: (030) 819-7561.
**Dusseldorf** — Cecillenallee 5. Telephone: (0211) 49 00 81.
**Frankfurt Am Main** — Siesmayerstrasse 21. Telephone: (0611) 74 0071; after hours call (0611) 74 50 04.
**Hamburg** — Alsterufer 27/28. Telephone: (040) 44 10 61.
**Munich** — Kö¢niginstrasse 5. Telephone: (089) 2 30 11.
**Stuttgart** — Urbanstrasse 7. Telephone: (0711) 21 02 21.

# Emergencies

■ **Help!**
  Hilfe!

■ **Police!**
  Polizei!

- **Fire!**
  Feuer!

- **I am ill.**
  Ich bin krank.

- **She is ill.**
  Sie ist krank.

- **He is ill.**
  Er ist krank.

- **Call a doctor right away.**
  Rufen Sie sofort einen Arzt.

- **Call an ambulance right away.**
  Rufen Sie sofort eine Ambulanz/einen Krankenwagen.

- **Take me/us to a doctor right away.**
  Bringen Sie mich/uns sofort zu einem Arzt.

- **Take me/us to a hospital right away.**
  Bringen Sie mich/uns sofort ins Krankenhaus.

- **Is there a doctor in the building?**
  Gibt es einen Arzt im Haus?

- **I cannot speak German. Please call this number for me.**
  Ich kann kein Deutsch. Bitte wählen Sie diese Nummer für mich.

# Emergency Telephone Numbers

When you arrive at your lodgings and check in, ask the clerk or manager for emergency telephone numbers. Of course, you'll feel foolish about making such a request even before you've seen your room or unpacked your bags, but no matter. Try out these phrases, and when you have the numbers, fill in the blanks of the *Emergency Telephone Numbers* box below. Or better still, ask the clerk to fill it in for you. If you show him or her the book with this official-looking box, your request won't appear so strange after all.

- **Emergency numbers belong in this box. Would you mind filling it in for me? Thank you.**

Notruf-Nummern hätte ich gerne in diesem Teil. Könnten Sie die bitte für mich einfüllen? Vielen Dank.

---

**Emergency Telephone Numbers— Notruf-Nummern**

Ambulance—Ambulanz: _____

Fire—Feuerwehr: _____

Police—Polizei: _____

---

# Asking for Help

- **Where is the nearest doctor?**

Wo findet man einen Arzt in der Nähe?

- **Where is the nearest hospital/clinic?**

Wo ist das nächste Krankenhaus/Klinik?

- **Where is the nearest first-aid station?**
Wo ist die nächste Erste-Hilfe-Station?

- **Where is the nearest pharmacy?**
Wo ist die nächste Apotheke?

- **Where is the nearest English-speaking doctor?**
Gibt es in der Nähe einen Arzt, der Englisch spricht?

- **Is there an English-speaking doctor here?**
Gibt es hier einen Arzt, der Englisch spricht?

- **Is there a hospital here with English-speaking doctors?**
Gibt es hier ein Krankenhaus mit Ärzten, die Englisch sprechen?

- **At what time can the doctor come?**
Wann kann der Arzt kommen?

- **What are the office hours?**
Wann sind die Sprechstunden?

- **Please PRINT the information. Thank you.**
Bitte geben Sie mir die Information in Druckschrift. Vielen Dank.

- **What is the doctor's name, address, and telephone number?**
Wie ist der Name, die Adresse, die Telefonnummer des Arztes?

- **Please show me where it is on this map.**
Bitte zeigen Sie mir auf der Karte, wo es ist.

- **Please show me on the map where we are now.**
Bitte zeigen Sie mir auf der Karte, wo wir sind.

- **Please draw a map/sketch for me.**
  Bitte zeichnen Sie es mir auf.

- **I cannot speak German. Please phone for me.**
  Ich kann kein Deutsch. Bitte rufen Sie für mich an.

- **Does anyone here speak English?**
  Spricht hier jemand Englisch?

- **I need an interpreter.**
  Ich brauche einen Dolmetscher.

# Numbers

0 — null
1 — eins
2 — zwei
3 — drei
4 — vier
5 — fünf
6 — sechs
7 — sieben
8 — acht
9 — neun
10 — zehn
11 — elf
12 — zwölf
13 — dreizehn
14 — vierzehn
15 — fünfzehn
16 — sechzehn
20 — zwanzig
21 — einundzwanzig
22 — zweiundzwanzig
30 — dreissig

31 — einunddreissig
32 — zweiunddreissig
40 — vierzig
41 — einundvierzig
42 — zweiundvierzig
50 — fünfzig
60 — sechzig
70 — siebzig
80 — achtzig
90 — neunzig
100 — hundert
101 — hunderteins
200 — zweihundert
300 — dreihundert
500 — fünfhundert
1000 — tausend
half — halb
quarter — viertel

# Section Four:
# Say It in French

# French Pronunciation

## General Rules

**1.** For most consonants, pronunciation in French and English is the same or similar. Exceptions are given below.
**2.** A *final* consonant in French is usually silent, as in *petit* (puh-tee).
**3.** The final e in a word of more than one syllable is silent, as in *petite* (puh-teet).
**4.** A normally silent final consonant is linked to the next word if the latter begins with a vowel. Example: *petit garçon* (puh-tee garçon), *petit enfant* (puh-teet enfant).

## Vowels

**a, à**  like **a** in marvel, but slightly shorter: *la dame, madame, la table*
**â**  like **a** in marvel but slightly drawn out: *pâté, pâle*
**e**  like **e** in verse
    —at the end of a one-syllable word: *me, que*
    —at the end of a syllable, as in *petit: pe tit*
**é**  like **a** in baby, but clipped, much shorter: *bébé, café*
**è, ê**  like **e** in set: *père, tête*
**i, î, y**  like the **i** in machine: *Michel, dîner, bicyclette*
**o**  —most often, an open **o** as in sort, port: *la porte, formidable*
    —closed **o** as in obey, pose, when followed by a single s: *la rose, la pose*
**ô**  closed **o,** as in obey: *le rôle*
**u**  a sound between **ee** and **oo** for which there is no equivalent in English. Round lips as if to whistle and say **ee**: *la tulipe*

# Vowel Combinations

**ai**   like **e** in set: *mauvais, faites*
**au, eau, aux, eaux** like **o** in **o**bey, but avoid any sound of
  u: *sauté, au revoir, château.* A final **x** linked to a
  succeeding vowel sounds like a **z**: *aux enfants*
**eu, eux, oeu, oeux** like **e** in serve: *fleur, soeur*
**ou**   like **oo** as in pool: *l'amour, vous, nous*
**oi**   like **wa** in **wa**ffle: *moi, voir*

# Nasal Sounds

**an, am, en, em, and, end, ant, ent** like the **a** in w**a**nt, but
  short, very nasal and without the sound of the **n** or
  **m**: *antique, manteau, enfant, tendre, employé, fervent.*
  Exception: -**en** at the end of a word is pronounced
  like the **in** in *bien*.
**in, im, ain, aim, yn, ym, ein** all pronounced like the **an** in
  **an**kle, **yan**kee: *vin, important, train, syndicat, sympa-
  thique, plein*
**on, om** like the **on** in d**on**'t; very short, very nasal: *pont,
  ombrelle*
**un, um** like the **oe** in d**oe**s, but nasal: *un, parfum.* (Do not
  sound the n or m.)

# Consonants and Combinations

**c**   like **k** before a, o, u, or a consonant: *café, cuisine,
  comique, client*
**c**   like **s** before e, i, y: *centre, cirque, bicyclette*
**ç**   like **s**: *français*
**ch**   like **sh**: *machine, chien*
**g**   like **g** in **g**ood, before a, o, u, or a consonant: *grand,
  gâteau, golfe, guerre*
  **gui**: **gee** as in **gee**se: *guide, guitare*
  **gue**: as in **gue**st: *guerre*

| | |
|---|---|
| **g** | like the **s** in pleasure before e, i, y: *gentille, gymnaste, giraffe* |
| **h** | not pronounced |
| **j** | like **s** in pleasure: *jardin* |
| **q** | always followed by **u**, pronounced like **k** in make<br>**que**: like **cu** in curtain: *que, quenelle*<br>**qui** (**kee**): *quiche*<br>**qua** (**kar**): *quart* |
| **s** | like **s** in set: *salade;* however, when it occurs between two vowels, it sounds like **z**: *cuisine* |
| **ss** | always like **s** in set: *pessimiste* |
| **t** | as in table; however, like **s** in set when in combinations: **tion, tiel, tial, tieux**: *nation, partiel* |
| **th** | like **t** in table: *mathémathiques* |
| **x** | pronounce as in English: *maxim;* however, in initial **ex** followed by a vowel, pronounce as **eggz**: *examen, exemple* |

# Basic Expressions in French

- **Yes**
  Oui

- **No**
  Non

- **Hello**
  Bonjour

- **Please**
  S'il vous plaît

- **Thank you**
  Merci

- **Excuse me**
  Excusez-moi

- **Pardon me**
  Pardonnez-moi

- **Good morning, Good afternoon, Good evening**
  Bonjour, Bonjour, Bonsoir

- **Good night, Good-bye**
  Bonne nuit, Au revoir

- **Where is the ladies'/men's room?**
  Où sont les toilettes pour dames/pour messieurs?

- **My name is _____.**
  Je m'appelle _____.

- **I am staying at _____.**
  Je suis à (l'hôtel) _____.

- **Can you help me?**
  Pouvez-vous m'aider?

- **Do you speak English?**
  Parlez-vous anglais?

- **Does anyone here speak English?**
  Y a-t-il quelqu'un ici qui parle anglais?

- **Can you find someone who speaks English?**
  Pouvez-vous trouver quelqu'un qui parle anglais?

- **I do not understand.**
  Je ne comprends pas.

- **Please speak slowly.**
  S'il vous plaît, parlez lentement.

- **Please repeat it.**
  Répétez, s'il vous plaît.

- **Please PRINT the directions.**
  Pouvez-vous m'indiquer le chemin par écrit et en caractères D'IMPRIMERIE?

- **Please PRINT it.**
  S'il vous plaît, écrivez-le en caractères D'IMPRIMERIE.

- **Please PRINT the name, address, and telephone number.**
  S'il vous plaît, écrivez en caractères D'IMPRIMERIE le nom, l'adresse, et le n° de téléphone.

- **Please show me on this map.**
  S'il vous plaît, montrez-moi sur cette carte.

- **Please show me on this map where I am.**
  S'il vous plaît, montrez-moi sur cette carte où je suis.

- **Please draw a map/sketch for me.**
  S'il vous plaît, dessinez-moi un plan.

- **Please call this number for me. Thank you.**
  S'il vous plaît, appelez ce n° de téléphone pour moi. Merci.

- **Where is the nearest _____?**
  Où est _____ le plus proche?

  - **hospital/clinic**
    hôpital/clinique
  - **first aid facility**
    poste de secours
  - **diet/health food/natural food restaurant**
    restaurant de diététique/de régime

- **Is the restaurant open/closed now?**
  Le restaurant est-il ouvert/fermé maintenant?

- **Please point to the days and hours it is open/closed.**
  S'il vous plaît, montrez-moi du doigt les heures et jours d'ouverture.

- **Monday**
  lundi

- **Tuesday**
  mardi

- **Wednesday**
  mecredi

- **Thursday**
  jeudi

- **Friday**
  vendredi

- **Saturday**
  samedi

- **Sunday**
  dimanche

- **a quarter past**
  et quart

- **half past**
  et demi

- **a quarter to**
  moins le quart

- **morning**
  matin

- **afternoon**
  après-midi

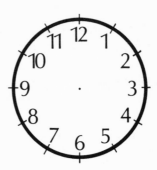

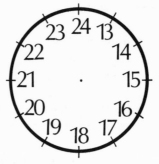

- **How much is this? Please write it down. (For a list of numbers, see page 223.)**
C'est combien? S'il vous plaît, écrivez-le-moi.

- **Do you have _____?**
Avez-vous _____?

- **I would like _____.**
J'aimerais _____.

- **Please give me _____.**
S'il vous plaît, donnez-moi _____.

# Dining Out in France

This section is divided into three parts. Part 1 includes a description of the hours for mealtimes, the available types of eating establishments, cover charges and tipping customs, plus some techniques of finding a restaurant and making reservations. Also, after finding a restaurant, there are questions included which you may need to ask, such as how to find a smoke-free spot. Part 2 gives some basic food lists arranged in breakfast, lunch, and dinner order. Part 3 contains a series of diet scenarios, each linked to specific health problems plus a scenario adaptable to the needs of travelers on special diets not covered in the more specific scenarios. Look them over now and check those items that will come in handy later.

## Part 1

### Mealtimes in France

Breakfast:   served between 7:30 and 10:30
Lunch:   served between 12:00 and 2:00
Dinner:   served between 7:30 and 10:00

Breakfast hours can be flexible, but lunch in France never starts before noon and dinner rarely before seven.

### Types of Eating Establishments in France

**Auberge** — a country inn that may have a restaurant attached to it.
**Brasserie** — a large establishment open very long hours and less formal than a restaurant. Combines the atmosphere of cafe and restaurant. Serves sandwiches as well as full meals.

**Buffet** — a restaurant at a railroad station.

**Café** — anything from a simple bar serving drinks, wine, coffee, hard-boiled eggs, simple ham sandwiches, and the like to a complete restaurant.

**Cafeteria** — a self-service establishment with flexible hours.

**Relais** — same as an *auberge*.

**Rôtisserie** — a restaurant whose specialty is broiling meat or fish to order in a section of the dining room.

**Routier** — a simple restaurant that can serve good food. It is usually found on highways and busy roads. Truck drivers frequent them, much as they do the simple diners on U.S. highways. You can recognize a *routier* by its red sign with blue circles.

**Salon de Thé** — a tea house. Pastries served with tea. Sometimes coffee and light sandwiches are also available.

# Tipping and Cover Charges in France

Tips range from 12 to 15 percent of the bill. Sometimes a tip is included in the charge. The menu may say this in very fine, easy-to-miss print. Look hard for: *service compris.* If you can't find a warning on the menu, that still doesn't mean that a tip hasn't been included. You must ask: *"Service compris?"* (Is the tip included in the bill?)

Sometimes there is also a cover charge (*couvert*). This information will appear on the menu, again sometimes in very fine print.

# Making Reservations in French Restaurants

Let the chef know you're coming and that you must observe a special diet. Ask your hotel manager or desk clerk to phone ahead for you. If you don't speak French, and your listeners don't speak English, simply point to the appropriate phrases.

Ask the desk clerk or hotel manager to read the following section before he or she phones for a reservation. To describe your needs, fill in the blanks with words and phrases selected from the "not permitted" list under your diet, the diet's scenario, the food lists, and the food preparation information in *Appendix 3*.

- **Can you recommend a good, but not too expensive restaurant?**
Pouvez-vous recommander un bon restaurant pas trop cher?

- **I have/she/he has a special problem and would like you to read the following:**
J'ai/elle a/il a un problème médical et j'aimerais que vous lisiez ceci.

- **I must ask a favor of you. I have/she/he has a medical problem and must observe a very special diet.**
Je dois vous demander une faveur. J'ai/elle a/il a un problème médical et doit observer un régime très strict.

- **Since I cannot speak French, may I ask you to phone the restaurant for me and explain the problem?**
Puisque je ne parle pas français, puis-je vous demander de téléphoner au restaurant et d'expliquer le problème?

- **May I ask you to do a favor for me/for us? Please phone this restaurant and make a reservation for a party of _____ for me for lunch/dinner. For today/tomorrow. For Monday/Tuesday/Wednesday/Thursday/Friday/Saturday/Sunday. At _____ o'clock.**
Puis-je/pouvons-nous vous demander une faveur? S'il vous plaît, téléphonez à ce restaurant et réservez pour un groupe de _____ pour moi pour déjeuner/dîner. Pour aujourd'hui/pour demain. Pour lundi/mardi/mecredi/jeudi/vendredi/samedi/dimanche. A _____ heure.

- **I/she/he cannot eat anything containing _____.**

Je/elle/il ne peut rien manger qui contient _____.

- **Eating anything containing _____ can cause serious illness.**

Une erreur peut avoir des conséquences graves.

- **Ask the maitre d' if he will be so kind as to arrange for simple substitutions in the dishes served to me.**

Demandez au maître d'hôtel s'il pourrait être assez aimable de faire substituer certains ingrédients simples dans le plat qu'on me servira.

- **For example, for lunch/dinner I would like _____ or _____.**

Par exemple, pour le déjeuner/le dîner j'aimerais _____ ou _____.

- **It should be _____ (method of preparation – see *Appendix* 3).**

Cela devrait être _____ (méthode de préparation).

- **It should not contain any _____.**

Cela ne devra contenir aucun _____.

- **Please ask for the name of the person with whom you are speaking. Write it down (PRINT it) for me. Thank you very much.**

S'il vous plaît, demandez le nom de la personne à qui vous parlez. Ecrivez-le-moi en caractères D'IMPRIMERIE. Je vous remercie beaucoup.

- **Please PRINT the name, address, and telephone number. Thank you.**

S'il vous plaît, écrivez en caractères D'IMPRIMERIE le nom, l'adresse, et le n° de téléphone. Merci.

After the call has been made, you can ask:

- **Have you made the reservation?**

Avez-vous réservé?

■ **Did they understand my/her/his problem?**
Ont-ils compris mon/son problème?

■ **Are they willing to arrange for special dishes?**
Peuvent-ils préparer des plats spéciaux?

You'll find these phrases helpful if you choose a restaurant on the spur of the moment.

■ **Are reservations necessary?**
Faut-il réserver?

■ **A table for _____, please. (See list of numbers on page 223.)**
Une table pour _____, s'il vous plaît.

■ **Do you have a nonsmoking section?**
Avez-vous un endroit non-fumeur?

■ **Please, can you seat me/us as far away from smokers as possible?**
S'il vous plaît, pourriez-vous me/nous mettre à une table le plus loin possible des fumeurs?

■ **I have/she/he has a serious allergy to smoke.**
J'ai/elle a/il a une grave allergie à la fumée.

■ **Where is the ladies'/men's room?**
Où sont les toilettes/les lavabos?

■ **Do you have _____?**
Avez-vous _____?

■ **I would like _____.**
J'aimerais _____.

- **Please give me _____.**
  S'il vous plaît, donnez-moi _____.
    - **glass of water (See pages 26–27 about water.)**
      un verre d'eau
    - **bottle of plain water/½ bottle of water**
      une bouteille/½ bouteille d'eau
    - **bottle of carbonated water**
      une bouteille d'eau gazeuse
    - **bottle of mineral water**
      une bouteille d'eau minérale
    - **fork/knife/spoon/napkin/straws**
      fourchette/couteau/cuillère/serviette/paille

# Part 2

The phrases and food lists in this section will be a big help in restaurants, supermarkets, and food stores. For a list of numbers, see page 223.

If you are on a low-sodium or low-potassium diet and are ordering or buying bottled water, consult the table on page 27 for the sodium and potassium levels of some popular brands.

## Breakfast

French breakfasts consist of tea or coffee with milk or cream, and bread, croissants or brioches served with butter, jelly or jam. Croissants are small, crescent-shaped rolls made of rich pastry—if you are on a low-fat diet, beware! Brioches are plump rolls made with less butter than the flaky croissants. These things together are sometimes known as the continental breakfast and are served to the exclusion of anything else; however, in hotels and restaurants that cater to an American clientele, you will find a more extensive breakfast menu.

# Fruit Juices – Jus de Fruit

Citrus fruit juices served in restaurants are generally freshly squeezed. Juices purchased in shops can be fresh, frozen, canned, or reconstituted from concentrate. If you have a preference, ask:

■ **Is this juice prepared from concentrate/from frozen juice?**
Est-ce que ce jus provient de concentré/de jus surgelé?

■ **I want only freshly squeezed orange/lemon juice.**
Je veux simplement une orange/un citron pressé.

■ **I want only canned/bottled fruit juice.**
Je veux simplement un jus de fruit en boîte/en bouteille.

■ **Do you have _____?**
Avez-vous _____?

■ **I would like _____.**
J'aimerais _____.

■ **Please give me _____.**
S'il vous plaît, donnez moi _____.

Select the juice you want from the following table, and ask for *jus de* _____ (the juice of _____).

# Fruit Juices

*English – French*
■ apple – pomme
■ apricot – abricot
■ grape – raisin

*French-English*
■ abricot – apricot
■ ananas – pineapple
■ citron – lemon

### English—French

- grapefruit—pamplemousse
- lemon—citron
- orange—orange
- pear—poire
- pineapple—ananas
- prune—pruneau
- tomato—tomate

### French—English

- orange—orange
- pamplemousse—grapefruit
- poire—pear
- pomme—apple
- pruneau—prune
- raisin—grape
- tomate—tomato

# Fruit—Fruit

### English—French

- apple—pomme
- applesauce—compote de pomme
- apricots—abricots
- avocado—avocat
- banana—banane
- blueberries—myrtilles
- cherries—cerises
- coconut—noix de coco
- dates—dattes
- figs—figues
- gooseberries—groseilles à maquereau
- grapefruit—pamplemousse
- grapes—raisin
- lemon—citron
- lime—citron vert
- melon—melon
- nectarine—brugnon
- olives—olives
- orange—orange
- peach—pêche
- pear—poire
- pineapple—ananas
- plum—prune
- pomegranates—grenades

### French—English

- abricots—apricots
- ananas—pineapple
- avocat—avocado
- banane—banana
- brugnon—nectarine
- cerises—cherries
- citron—lemon
- citron vert—lime
- clémentine—tangerine (small)
- coing—quince
- compote de pomme—applesauce
- dattes—dates
- figues—figs
- fraises—strawberries
- fraises des bois—wild strawberries
- framboises—raspberries
- grenades—pomegranates
- groseilles—red currants
- groseilles à maquereau—gooseberries
- mandarine—tangerine
- melon—melon
- myrtilles—blueberries
- noix—walnuts

*(continued on next page)*

**Dining Out**

**French**

# Fruit — Fruit (continued)

*English — French*
- prunes — pruneaux
- raisins — raisins secs
- raspberries — framboises
- red currants — groseilles
- quince — coing
- strawberries — fraises
- strawberries, wild — fraises des bois
- tangerine — mandarine or clémentine (small)
- walnuts — noix
- watermelon — pastèque

*French — English*
- noix de coco — coconut
- olives — olives
- pamplemousse — grapefruit
- pastèque — watermelon
- pêche — peach
- poire — pear
- pomme — apple
- prune — plum
- pruneaux — prunes
- raisin — grapes
- raisins secs — raisins

Now that you've had your fruit juice and/or fruit, you might want to go on to something more substantial and nutritious for breakfast. If you are taking breakfasts at your hotel, speak with the manager or the maitre d' the day or evening before your first morning meal. Try these phrases:

- **May I ask a special favor of you?**

Puis-je vous demander une faveur spéciale?

- **Would it be possible to have _____ for breakfast?**

Pour le petit déjeuner, serait-il possible d'avoir _____?

Select something from the following lists of breakfast foods, but keep it simple. If necessary, show your WALLET CARD; it will lend authority to your request. If your food must be prepared in a certain way, point to the appropriate phrases *(Appendix 3)*. Better still, put it all down on paper before you approach the maitre d'. PRINT it! Of course, you'll feel a little silly and embarrassed the very first time you flash your WALLET CARD and make a special request. Who wouldn't? But keep in mind that the hotel staff is anxious to make your stay a comfortable one. The important thing is to be polite and friendly when making your request. After you've tried it once, you'll become an old hand at it. Okay, let's get back to breakfast.

# Cereals – Céréales

Like cereals? Remember, while cold cereals are a staple in French stores, you'll find them *only* in hotels and restaurants catering predominantly to an American clientele. Cold cereals can be requested or bought under their English names; no translation is necessary. So, if your taste runs to cornflakes, and you want to find out if there are any on hand, all you need to say is *"Avez-vous des cornflakes?"*

## Hot Cereals

Hot cereal for breakfast in France? When this book went to press, it was a rare item, but by now it may be on some breakfast menus. Again, if you are staying at a large hotel that caters to Americans, you are more likely to find hot cereal, or at least have a special order for it filled. Try this list when ordering:
- barley—céréale d'orge
- bran—son
- buckwheat—céréale de sarrasin (blé noir)
- oatmeal—céréale aux flocons d'avoine
- rice—riz (If all you want is a bowl of hot rice with milk for breakfast, you shouldn't have any problem; every chef stocks rice.)
- rye—céréale de seigle
- soy—soja
- wheat cereal—céréale au blé
- wild rice—riz sauvage
- wheat germ—germe de blé

If the waiter or chef says *"oui,"* then you might want to add:

■ **Please cook it in unsalted water.**
S'il vous plaît, faites le cuire dans de l'eau non salée.

■ **Don't put any _____ in it.**
Ne mettez aucun _____ dedans.

■ **Please put some _____ in it.**
S'il vous plaît, mettez du/de la _____ dedans.

If your digestive problem requires a highly refined cereal,. ask:

■ **Do you have any refined cereals suitable for babies?**
Avez-vous des céréales pour bébé (moulues très fines)?

# Bread — Pain

If you are planning to stay at a hotel for any length of time or dine frequently at one restaurant, you can ask the maitre d' to get salt-free bread for you:

■ **I am on a special salt-free diet.**
Je suis un régime spécial sans sel.

■ **Can you get salt-free bread for me?**
Pouvez-vous m'obtenir du pain sans sel?.

French bakeries produce many varieties of white bread: those flaky, butter-rich rolls, croissants, and their slightly less buttery cousins, brioches. You might prefer something like our melba toast—*biscottes* or *biscottes sans sel* (without salt).
How do you want your bread or rolls?

■ **Please toast the bread.**
S'il vous plaît, faites griller le pain.

■ **Please warm the _____.**
S'il vous plaît, chauffez le_____.

# Eggs — Oeufs

• fried—au plat/sur le plat
• hard-boiled—dur
• plain omelet—omelette nature
• poached—poché

- scrambled—brouillé
- soft-boiled—à la coque

# Dairy Products—Produits Laitiers

If you are in a small village and have doubts about pasteurization and refrigeration, you may want to ask about milk, cheese or other dairy products.

■ **Is it pasteurized?**
  Est-ce pasteurisé?

■ **Has it been refrigerated?**
  Etait-ce réfrigéré?

- butter—beurre
- sweet (unsalted) butter—beurre doux or sans sel
- margarine—margarine
- diet (low calorie)—de régime

### Cheese—Fromage
France is a country of cheeses, and more than 300 are available.

If you're worried about calories and fat in cheese, ask about what's sometimes listed as the % MG on cheese labels, the percentage of *matières grasses* (fat) in DM (dry matter).

■ **I would like a cheese with a minimum of fat. What do you recommend?**
  Je voudrais un fromage dont le pourcentage de matières grasses soit très faible. Que me recommandez-vous?

Are you looking for a low-salt cheese? Ask:

■ **I would like a salt-free cheese or a cheese very low in salt. What do you recommend?**
  Je voudrais un fromage sans sel ou avec très peu de sel. Que me recommandez-vous?

■ **Is it a very salty cheese?**
Est-ce un fromage très salé?

■ **Can you recommend a cheese not too salty/not too fat?**
Pouvez-vous recommander un fromage pas trop
salé/très maigre?

■ **Do you have a cheese with no salt—a gruyère/a gouda?**
Avez-vous un fromage sans sel—un gruyère sans
sel/un gouda?

■ **Do you have a _gaperon_ (a cheese with peppercorns and 30
percent fat) or a very lean cheese like it (with a minimum of fat)?**
Avez-vous un gaperon ou un fromage très maigre
comme le gaperon?

■ **Is this cheese made with whole milk?**
Est-ce un fromage au lait entier?

■ **Is this cheese made with skim milk?**
Est-ce un fromage au lait écrémé?

■ **Is this cheese made with part skim milk?**
Est-ce un fromage ½ écrémé (demi-écrémé)?

You should also know if an extra dose of cream has been
added to your cheese during the manufacturing process:

■ **Is it a double cream?**
Est-ce un double crème?

Or, a super dose of cream may have been added:

■ **Is it a triple cream?**
Est-ce un triple crème?

■ **What percentage of fat does it contain?**
Quel est le pourcentage de matières grasses?

■ **Please write it down. Thank you.**
S'il vous plaît, écrivez-le-moi. Merci.

■ **Do you have a cheese with less than 40 percent fat that is salt-free?**
Avez-vous un ou des fromages à 40% ou moins, sans sel?

■ **Do you have cottage cheese?**
Avez-vous un fromage blanc?
  • without cream—sans crème
  • salt-free—sans sel

## Yogurt—Yaourt/Yoghourt
■ **Do you have yogurt that is _____?**
Avez-vous un yaourt/yoghourt _____?
  • made with whole milk—au lait entier
  • made with skim milk—au lait écrémé
  • containing fruit—aux fruits
  • plain (no fruit)—nature
  • without sugar or sweetening—sans sucre ou substance pour sucrer

## Cream—Crème
Ordinary sweet cream is *crème* in France. A popular cream is called *crème fraîche;* it is similar to sour cream in appearance but not in taste. *Crème fraîche* is used in recipes and as a topping for fruits. *Crème aigre* is our sour cream, and it is not as popular as in this country. If you use none of the above but prefer a nondairy creamer, you're probably out of luck in France, because it is rare there. However, you might try restaurants by asking for *un produit non latier—imitation de lait (de crème).*

## Milk—Lait
  • buttermilk—babeurre
  • condensed milk—condensé, avec sucre

183

- evaporated skim milk—lait écrémé condensé sans sucre (évaporé)
- evaporated whole milk—lait entier condensé sans sucre (évaporé)
- fresh skim milk—lait frais écrémé
- fresh whole milk—lait frais ordinaire
- homogenized—homogénéisé
- not homogenized—pas homogénéisé
- kefir—kéfir
- pasteurized—pasteurisé
- powdered skim milk—lait en poudre écrémé
- powdered whole milk—lait en poudre entier

## Spreads

- honey—miel
- jam—confiture
- jelly—gelée
- marmalade—marmelade
- peanut butter (never served in restaurants and available only in specialty shops)—beurre de cacahuète/beurre d'arachide

## Beverages — Boissons

- chocolate (cocoa)—chocolat
- coffee—café
- decaffeinated coffee—café décaffeiné
- espresso coffee (very strong stuff)—café express
- herb tea—tisane/infusion
- tea—thé

For an additional listing of beverages, see pages 193–195.

# Lunch and Dinner

Worried about preparation? Consult *Appendix 3: French Food Preparation.*

If you are curious about the meat in a dish on a menu, ask:

- **What kind of meat is this?**
Quelle sorte de viande est-ce?

- **Please show me on this list.**
S'il vous plaît, montrez-moi sur cette liste.

- **I would like _____.**
J'aimerais _____.

- very lean—très maigre
- without fat—sans gras
- beef—boeuf
- chicken—poulet
- lamb—mouton (young lamb [*agneau*] is more tender.)
- pork—porc
- turkey—dinde, young turkey—dindonneau
- veal—veau

Meats are cut differently in France than in the United States. Therefore, the names of cuts listed below are only approximations. Also, meats, by law, are much leaner than they are in the United States.

Here are some cuts of meat, listed by category—beef, lamb, pork, poultry, veal, and variety meats.

## Cuts of Meat

*English—French*
**Beef—*Boeuf***
- beef, very lean—boeuf très maigre
- beefsteak—biftek
- bottom round—sous noix
- chuck—macreuse, côtes découvertes
- flank steak—bavette
- liver (lean, but *high* in cholesterol)—foie
- plate ribs—plates côtes
- plate skirt steak—tendron

*French—English*
**Boeuf—Beef**
- bavette—flank steak
- biftek—beefsteak
- boeuf très maigre—very lean beef
- côtes découvertes—chuck
- filet de boeuf—tenderloin
- foie—liver
- gîte à la noix—top round
- plates côtes—plate ribs
- romsteck—rump

*(continued on next page)*

# Cuts of Meat (continued)

## English—French
**Beef—*Boeuf* (continued)**
- roast beef—rosbif
- rump—romsteck
- tenderloin—filet de boeuf
- top round—gîte à la noix
- tripe—tripes

**Lamb—*Mouton*;**
**Young Lamb—*Agneau***
- chop—côte or côtelette
- leg—gigot
- loin chops—côtes de filet
- loin roast—selle
- rib—côtelette première
- shank—collet
- shoulder—épaule

**Pork—*Porc***
- ham—jambon
  - ham, fresh—jambon frais
  - ham, smoked— jambon fumé
- pork chops, pork cutlets— côtelettes de porc
- suckling pig—porcelet, cochon de lait

**Poultry—*Volaille***
- capon—poussin
- chicken—poulet
  - breast—blanc de poulet or filet de poulet
  - leg—cuisse de poulet
  - roast chicken—poulet rôti
- duck—canard; duckling— caneton

## French—English
**Boeuf—Beef**
- rosbif—roast beef
- soux noix—bottom round
- tendron—plate skirt steak
- tripes—tripe

**Mouton—Lamb;**
**Agneau—Young Lamb**
- collet—shank
- côte—chop
- côtelette—chop
- côtelette première—rib
- côtes de filet—loin chops
- épaule—shoulder
- gigot—leg
- selle—loin roast

**Porc—Pork**
- cochon de lait—suckling pig
- côtelettes de porc—pork chops, pork cutlets
- jambon—ham
- jambon frais—fresh ham
- jambon fumé—smoked ham
- porcelet—suckling pig

**Volaille—Poultry**
- blanc de dinde—turkey breast
- blanc de poulet—chicken breast
- caille—quail
- canard—duck
- canard sauvage—wild duck
- caneton—duckling

## English—French

- duck, wild—canard sauvage
- goose—oie
- guinea hen—pintade
- hen—poule
- partridge—perdreau, perdrix
- pheasant—faisan
- pigeon—pigeon
- quail—caille
- squab—pigeon, pigeonneau
- turkey—dinde, young turkey—dindonneau
    - breast—blanc de dinde or filet de dinde
    - leg—cuisse de dinde
    - roast turkey—dinde rôti

## French—English

- cuisse de dinde—turkey leg
- cuisse de poulet—chicken leg
- dinde—turkey
- dinde rôti—roast turkey
- dindonneau—young turkey
- faisan—pheasant
- filet de dinde—turkey breast
- oie—goose
- perdreau—partridge
- perdrix—partridge
- pigeon—pigeon, squab
- pigeonneau—squab
- pintade—guinea hen
- poule—hen
- poulet—chicken
- poulet rôti—roast chicken
- poussin—capon

## Veal—*Veau*

- cutlets—escalope
- leg—jarret
- loin—côtelette première
- rib—côte or côtelette
- shank—jarret or rouelle
- shoulder—épaule

## *Veau*—Veal

- côte—rib
- côtelette—rib
- côtelette première—loin
- épaule—shoulder
- escalope—cutlet
- jarret—leg, shank
- rouelle—shank

## Other Meats and Variety Meats

- bacon—bacon or lard maigre (poitrine fumée)
- blood sausage—boudin noir
- brains—cervelle
- goat/kid—chèvre
- hare—lièvre
- kidneys—rognons

- bacon—bacon
- boudin noir—blood sausage
- cervelle—brains
- chèvre—goat/kid
- langue—tongue
- lapin—rabbit
- lièvre—hare

*(continued on next page)*

Dining Out

French

# Cuts of Meat (continued)

*English—French*

**Other Meats and Variety Meats (continued)**

- mutton—mouton
- oxtail—queue de boeuf
- pig's feet—pieds de porc
- rabbit—lapin
- rabbit, wild—lièvre
- salami—saucisson
- sausages—saucisses (mergues: a North African spiced sausage)
- sweetbreads—ris de veau
- tongue—langue
- venison—venaison

*French—English*

- mergues—a North African spiced sausage
- mouton—mutton
- pieds de porc—pig's feet
- queue de boeuf—oxtail
- ris de veau—sweetbreads
- rognons—kidneys
- saucisses—sausages
- saucisson—salami
- venaison—venison

# Fish—Poisson and Shellfish—Coquillages

- **What kind of fish is this?**
  Quelle sorte de poisson est-ce?

- **Please show me on this list.**
  S'il vous plaît, montrez-moi sur cette liste.

- **Is it fresh?**
  Est-ce du poisson frais?

- **Has it been frozen and thawed?**
  Est-ce du poisson surgelé et dégivré?

- **Fillet it for me, please.**
  Faites-le-moi en filet, s'il vous plaît.

- **Do you have _____?**
  Avez-vous _____?

- **I would like _____.**
  J'aimerais _____.

- **Please give me _____.**
  S'il vous plaît, donnez-moi _____.

# Fresh and Saltwater Fish

## English—French

- anchovy—anchois
- angler (tilefish)—baudroie (lotte)
- bass—bar or loup
- brill—barbue
- carp—carpe
- clam (the French version)—palourde
- cod—morue (cabillaud)
- cod, fresh—cabillaud (morue)
- crab—crabe
- crab (the French version)—araignée (long legs)
- crawfish—langouste
- deep-fried little fish—friture
- eel—anguille
- gudgeon (freshwater)—goujon
- gurnard mullet—grondin
- haddock—aiglefin
- hake—colin (merlu)
- hake, small—merlu (colin)
- halibut—flétan
- herring—hareng
- lemon sole—limande
- lobster—homard
- mackerel—maquereau
- mixed seafood (shellfish)—fruits de mer
- mussels—moules

## French—English

- aiglefin—haddock
- anchois—anchovy
- anguille—eel
- araignée—a French long-legged crab
- bar—bass
- barbue—brill
- baudroie—angler (tilefish)
- bigorneau—periwinkle
- brochet—pike
- cabillaud—fresh cod
- calmar—squid
- carpe—carp
- carrelet—plaice (a variety of flounder)
- colin—hake
- crabe—crab
- daurade—sea bream or porgy
- encornet—small squid
- éperlan—smelt
- espadon—swordfish
- flétan—halibut
- friture—deep-fried little fish
- fruits de mer—mixed seafood (shellfish)
- goujon—gudgeon (freshwater)
- grondin—gurnard mullet
- hareng—herring
- homard—lobster

*(continued on next page)*

# Fresh and Saltwater Fish
(continued)

*English—French*
- octopus—poulpe
- oyster—huître
- periwinkle—bigorneau
- pike—brochet
- plaice (a variety of flounder)—carrelet
- porgy (sea bream)—daurade
- salmon—saumon
  - salmon, smoked—saumon fumé
- salmon trout—truite saumonée
- sardines—sardines
- sea bass—loup de mer
- sea bream (porgy)—daurade
- sea urchin—oursin
- skate—raie
- smelt—éperlan
- sole—sole
- sole (the French version)—plie
- squid—calmar
- squid, small—encornet
- swordfish—espadon
- tilefish (angler)—baudroie or lotte
- trout—truite
- tuna—thon
- turbot—turbot
- whiting—merlan

*French—English*
- huître—oyster
- langouste—crawfish (crayfish)
- limande—lemon sole
- lotte—angler (tilefish)
- loup—bass
- loup de mer—sea bass
- maquereau—mackerel
- merlan—whiting
- merlu—small hake
- morue—cod
- moule—mussel
- oursin—sea urchin
- palourde—a French clam
- plie—the French version of sole
- poulpe—octopus
- raie—skate
- sardines—sardines
- saumon—salmon
- saumon fumé—smoked salmon
- sole—sole
- thon—tuna
- truite—trout
- truite saumonée—salmon trout
- turbot—turbot

# Vegetables — Légumes

- **Do you have _____?**
  Avez-vous _____?

- **I would like _____.**
  J'aimerais _____.

- **Please give me _____.**
  S'il vous plaît, donnez-moi _____.

# Vegetables

*English—French*
- artichokes—artichauts
- asparagus—asperges
- avocado—avocat
- beans—haricots
  - kidney beans—
    haricots à écosser
  - string beans—
    haricots verts
  - white kidney beans—
    haricots blancs
- broccoli (very rare in
  France)—broccoli
- brussels sprouts—
  choux de Bruxelles
- cabbage—chou
  - red cabbage—
    chou rouge
- capers—câpres
- carrots—carottes
- cauliflower—chou-fleur
- celery—céleri
- celery root—céleri-rave
- chervil—cerfeuil
- chick-peas—pois
  chiches
- chicory—chicorée
- chives—ciboulette
- corn (not common)—
  maïs
- cucumber—concombre

*French—English*
- aïl—garlic
- artichaut—artichoke
- asperges—asparagus
- aubergine—eggplant
- avocat—avocado
- blette—Swiss chard
- broccoli—broccoli
- câpres—capers
- carottes—carrots
- céleri—celery
- céleri-rave—celery root
- cerfeuil—chervil
- champignons (de Paris,
  bolet, cèpe, girolle,
  morille, mousseron)—
  mushrooms
- chicorée—chicory
- chou—cabbage
- chou-fleur—cauliflower
- chou rouge—red cabbage
- choux de Bruxelles—
  brussels sprouts
- ciboulette—chives
- coeurs de palmier—
  palm hearts
- concombre—cucumber
- cornichons—gherkins
- courgette—zucchini
- cresson—watercress
- échalottes—shallots

*(continued on next page)*

# Vegetables   (continued)

## English—French

- eggplant—aubergine
- endives—endives
- fennel—fenouil
- garlic—aïl
- gherkins—cornichons
- Jerusalem artichokes—topinambours
- leeks—poireaux
- lentils—lentilles
- lettuce—laitue
- lima beans—fèves
- mushrooms—champignons (de Paris, bolet, cèpe, girolle, morille, mousseron)
- onions—oignons
- palm hearts—coeurs de palmier
- parsley—persil
- parsnips—navets
- peas—petits pois
- peppers—poivrons
- potato—pomme de terre
- pumpkin—potiron
- radishes—radis
- shallots—échalottes
- sorrel—oseille
- spinach—épinards
- sweet peppers—poivrons doux
- sweet potato—patate douce
- Swiss chard—blette
- tomato—tomate
- truffles—truffes
- turnip—navet
- watercress—cresson
- zucchini—courgette

## French—English

- endives—endives
- épinards—spinach
- fenouil—fennel
- fèves—lima beans
- haricots à écosser—kidney beans
- haricots blancs—white kidney beans
- haricots vert—string beans
- laitue—lettuce
- lentilles—lentils
- maïs—corn
- navet—turnip
- oignons—onions
- oseille—sorrel
- patate douce—sweet potato
- persil—parsley
- petits pois—peas
- poireaux—leeks
- pois chiches—chick-peas
- poivron—pepper
- poivron doux—sweet pepper
- pomme de terre—potato
- potiron—pumpkin
- radis—radishes
- tomate—tomato
- topinambours—Jerusalem artichokes
- truffes—truffles

# Pasta – Pâtes

■ **Please cook it in unsalted water.**
S'il vous plaît, faites-le cuire dans de l'eau non salée.

■ **Was this cooked in salted water?**
Était-ce cuit dans l'eau salée?

■ **Please ask the chef to check the label on the container. Does it contain any _____?**
S'il vous plait, demandez au chef de regarder l'étiquette de la boîte. Cela contient-il du/de la _____?
  - egg—oeuf
  - salt—sel
  - sugar—sucre
  - sweetening—agent sucreur

### Pasta Products
- macaroni—macaroni
- made with white flour—farine blanche complète
- made with whole wheat flour—farine complète
- noodles—nouilles
- spaghetti—spaghetti
- spinach noodles—nouilles aux épinards
- vermicelli—vermicelle

# Nonalcoholic Beverages – Boissons non Alcooliques

■ **Do you have _____?**
Avez-vous _____?

■ **I would like _____.**
J'aimerais _____.

■ **Please give me _____.**
S'il vous plaît, donnez-moi _____.

- black coffee—café noir
- chocolate or cocoa (hot)—chocolat
- Coca-Cola—Coca-Cola
- coffee with cream—café crème
- coffee with milk—café au lait
- espresso—café express
- iced coffee—café glacé
- lemonade, bottled—limonade
- lemonade, freshly squeezed—citron pressé
- mineral water—eau minéral
- orangeade, bottled—orangeade
- syrup—sirop*
- tea—thé
    - thé au lait—tea with milk
    - thé citron—tea with lemon
    - thé nature—regular tea
- tonic water—tonique

For additional listings of nonalcoholic beverages, see page 184.

# Wines — Vins

- Alsatian—Alsace
- Bordeaux—Bordeaux
- burgundy—Bourgogne
- champagne—Champagne
- Côte du Rhône (red)—Côte du Rhône
- Loire—Loire
- Provence—Provence
- red—rouge
- rosé—rosé
- sparkling—mousseux
- white—blanc

*Sirop: Choice of many different fruit and herb-flavored (mint, anise) syrups which are mixed with water.

## Alcoholic Drinks —
## Boissons Alcooliques

- Armagnac (brandy)—Armagnac
- beer—bière
    - light—bière blonde
    - dark—bière brune
- bourbon—bourbon
- brandy—fine
- cider—cidre
- cognac (brandy)—cognac
- gin—gin
- liqueur—liqueur
- port—porto
- rum—rhum
- sherry—sherry
- vodka—vodka
- whiskey—whiskey

# Part 3

## The Low-Sodium (Low-Salt) Diet

The following list of "not permitted" items may vary from the list of foods your physician has instructed you to avoid. To make the list easier for others to read, cross out the items that do not apply to you and write in, PRINTING LEGIBLY, any other items you must avoid. Select them from the food lists on pages 175–194.

To make sure your food and beverages are prepared properly, consult *Appendix 3: French Food Preparation.* Use it together with other appropriate pages when ordering meals.

Keep in mind these hidden sodium sources: baked goods may be made with baking powder (sodium bicarbonate) rather than yeast. Ask:

■ **Is this made with yeast?**

Cela est-il fait avec du levain (levure de boulanger)?

■ **Is this made with baking powder/baking soda?**

Cela est-il fait avec de la levure chimique/du bicarbonate de soude?

Beware also that antacids, like Alka Seltzer, and other
indigestion aids may contain sodium bicarbonate or other
sodium compounds. Before you go abroad, ask your
physician to suggest a low-sodium antacid to take along.
If you must buy an antacid in France, here's the French for
sodium bicarbonate or bicarbonate of soda: *bicarbonate
de soude.* Other sodium compounds will have the word
*sodium* in them. It's the same word in French and English
or the symbol for sodium, which is Na, will be used. Look
for it on labels. Also, if you must keep to a diet of less
than 800 milligrams of sodium a day, don't use softened
water. Ask:

■ **Does this water/the water in the hotel pass through a filter
that softens it/removes the hard minerals?**

Est-ce que cette eau/l'eau de l'hôtel est filtrée pour
l'adoucir/pour éliminer les minéraux?

Check the labels on bottled water and mineral water
for sodium content. If the label does not contain a chemical
analysis, use the table on page 27 as a guideline.
So far all you've read is *avoid, not permitted, beware,*
and you're wondering what you *can* eat or drink in France
and still stick to your diet. Unfortunately, your diet scenario
sounds pretty negative too, but don't let that frighten you.
Take a look at the extensive food lists in *Part 2* of this
section, pages 175–194. If you can't order from the menu
the waiter gives you, ask for items on these foods lists.
Combine your selections with help from *Appendix 3:
French Food Preparation* and the diet scenario that
follows for a satisfying meal, one custom-made to your
specifications.
Mayonnaise served in restaurants is almost always
homemade, so, if you would like a portion without salt,
ask:

■ **I have a special favor to ask of you.**

J'ai une faveur spéciale à vous demander.

- **Can you prepare a portion/serving of mayonnaise for me without salt?**

  Pourriez-vous me préparer une mayonnaise faite sans sel?

  Another special, salt-free dish you might request is steamed potatoes. It is a popular side order in French restaurants and can be prepared without salt. Ask:

- **May I have a serving of steamed potatoes, plain, without salt?**

  Puis-je avoir des pommes vapeur, toutes simples, sans sel?

  If you want your salad without dressing, ask:

- **Can you serve the salad plain, without dressing?**

  Pouvez-vous m'apporter la salade sans vinaigrette?

Or, you might want the salad dressing served separately, on the side!

- **Can you serve the salad dressing separately, on the side?**

  Pouvez-vous m'apporter la vinaigrette à part?

  To be sure your butter is unsalted, ask:

- **May I have a serving of unsalted butter?**

  Puis-je avoir du beurre non salé?

---

# Foods Not Permitted — Aliments Interdits

- anything baked with baking powder or with baking soda—tout ce qui est fait avec de la levure chimique ou du bicarbonate de soude
- bacon drippings—saindoux/ bacon
- baking soda—bicarbonate de soude
- bouillon—bouillon

*(continued on next page)*

# Foods Not Permitted – Aliments Interdits (continued)

- broth—consommé
- canned fish—poisson en conserve
- canned meat—viande en conserve
- canned tomatoes—tomates en conserve
- canned vegetables— légumes en conserve
- capers—câpres
- catsup—ketchup
- celery salt—sel de céleri
- cheese—fromage
- chive—ciboulette
- cold cuts—charcuterie
- condensed milk—lait condensé
- gherkins—cornichons
- gravy—jus
- horseradish—raifort
- instant or frozen potatoes— pommes de terre instantanées ou surgelées
- margarine—margarine
- mayonnaise—mayonnaise
- meat sauce—jus de viande
- milk—lait
- monosodium glutamate (MSG)—glutamate monosodique
- mustard—moutarde
- salt—sel
- salted butter—beurre salé
- salted salad dressing— vinaigrette salée
- sausage—saucisse
- sodium preservatives— sodium comme agent de conservation
- soy sauce—sauce de soja
- tomato puree—purée de tomate
- tomato sauce—sauce tomate ou concentrée

# The Low-Sodium (Low-Salt) Scenario

If you can't pronounce the French, point to appropriate phrases. For some sample replies to your questions, turn to *Appendix 3: French Food Preparation* and show it to your respondent.

- **I have a reservation. My name is _____.**
  J'ai réservé. Je m'appelle _____.

- **Please tell the manager I am here.**
  S'il vous plaît, dites au directeur que je suis ici.

■ **The manager knows about the special service I need because of a medical problem.**

Le directeur est au courant d'un service spécial qu'il doit me rendre à cause d'un problème médical.

■ **Does anyone here speak English?**

Y a-t-il quelqu'un ici qui parle anglais?

■ **I/she/he must follow a special diet.**

Je/elle/il doit suivre un régime spécial.

■ **All food and drink must be completely salt-free.**

Tout—nourritures, boissons—doit être absolument sans sel.

■ **Everything must be prepared without the items on this list.**

Aucun des ingrédients de cette liste ne doivent figurer dans la préparation de ce que je peux manger.

■ **A mistake can cause serious illness.**

Une erreur peut avoir des conséquences graves.

■ **Does this dish contain any salt?**

Ce plat contient-il du sel?

■ **Does this dish contain anything on this list?**

Y a-t-il un ou plusieurs des ingrédients de cette liste dans ce plat?

■ **Can you prepare this dish without salt?**

Pouvez-vous préparer ce plat sans sel?

■ **Can you prepare this dish without any of the items on this list?**

Pouvez-vous préparer ce plat sans aucun des ingrédients de cette liste?

■ **Show me on the menu which dishes you can prepare without salt.**

Montrez-moi sur le menu quels plats vous pouvez préparer sans sel.

■ **Show me on the menu which dishes you can prepare without any of the items on this list?**

Indiquez-moi sur le menu lesquels des plats vous pouvez préparer sans aucun des ingrédients de cette liste.

■ **Which dishes on the menu are salt-free?**

Quels plats sur le menu ne contiennent pas de sel?

■ **Are there any dishes on the menu that do not contain ingredients forbidden to me?**

Y a-t-il sur le menu des plats qui ne contiennent aucun des ingrédients qui me sont interdits?

■ **Are the tomatoes in this dish fresh, frozen or canned? (Waiter, please point to the right word.)**

Les tomates dans ce plat sont-elles fraîches, surgelées ou en conserve? (Garçon, s'il vous plaît, indiquez-moi le mot correct.)

■ **Is the pasta cooked in salted water?**

Les pâtes sont-elles cuites à l'eau salée?

■ **Can you prepare a serving of pasta for me, cooked in unsalted water?**

Pouvez-vous me servir une portion de pâtes cuites à l'eau sans sel?

■ **Are the potatoes/vegetables cooked in salted water?**

Les pommes de terre/légumes sont-ils cuits à l'eau salée?

- **Can you prepare potatoes/vegetables for me, cooked in unsalted water?**
  Pouvez-vous me servir des pommes de terre/des légumes cuits à l'eau non salée?

- **If you are not sure, please tell me/ask the chef/the maitre d'.**
  Si vous n'êtes pas sûr, s'il vous plaît, dites-le-moi/demandez au chef/au maître d'hôtel.

- **I would like to speak to the chef/the maitre d'.**
  Je voudrais parler au chef/au maître d'hôtel.

- **Can you prepare something simple for me in your kitchen that is salt-free? For example, baked or broiled fish; steak; steamed, boiled, or mashed potatoes; fresh, cooked, unsalted vegetables?**
  Pouvez-vous me préparer quelque chose de simple à la cuisine, *absolument sans sel*? Par exemple, du poisson au four ou grillé; ou un steak grillé; avec des pommes vapeur, ou à l'anglaise ou en purée; des légumes frais, dans de l'eau sans sel.

- **Do you have a microwave oven/a pressure cooker?**
  Avez-vous un four à micro-ondes/une marmite à pression?

  (If the answer is *yes,* then ask:)

- **Can you prepare a single portion of _____, plain/without seasoning/gravy/sauce/salt?**
  Pouvez-vous préparer une portion de _____ très simple, sans assaisonnement/jus/sauce/sel?

- **A mistake has been made. This is not what I ordered.**
  Il y a une erreur. Ce n'est pas ce que j'ai commandé.

# The Diabetic Diet

Your physician has outlined a personal diet and probably shown you how to select balanced meals using a system of food exchanges. The phrases in this section will help you identify dishes on a menu that contain added sweetening. If you must also observe a low-fat diet, refer to the low-fat and low-cholesterol phrases on page 207.

**Caution:** If you must take an antacid, be sure to read the information on page 15 about the sugar content of many popular antacids.

To make sure your food and drink are properly prepared, consult *Appendix 3: French Food Preparation.* Use it together with other appropriate pages when ordering meals.

Check the "not permitted" list. To make it easier for others to read, cross out the items that do not apply to you, and add, PRINTING LEGIBLY, the things you cannot have. Select your additions from the food lists on pages 175–194.

The use of synthetic sweeteners of any type is forbidden in the preparation of food products in France. Therefore, diet sodas are unknown. Saccharin, however, can be obtained at any pharmacy without a prescription. If you sweeten your food or beverages with saccharin, you must carry your own when dining out.

# Foods Not Permitted— Aliments Interdits

- barley syrup—sirop d'orge, orgeat
- butter—beurre
- condensed milk—lait condensé
- corn sweetener— agent sucreur contenu dans le maïs
- dextrose—dextrose
- fats—gras
- fructose—fructose
- honey—miel
- jam—confiture
- jelly—gelée de fruits
- lard—saindoux
- maltose—maltose
- margarine—margarine
- marmalade— marmelade
- molasses—mélasse
- oils—huiles
- rice syrup—sirop de riz
- sugar—sucre
- syrup—sirop

# The Diabetic Scenario

If you cannot pronounce the French, point to the appropriate phrases. For some sample replies to your questions, turn to *Appendix 3: French Food Preparation* and show it to your respondent.

■ **I have a reservation. My name is _____.**

J'ai réservé. Je m'appelle _____.

■ **Please tell the manager I am here.**

S'il vous plaît, dites au directeur que je suis ici.

■ **The manager knows about the special service I need because of a medical problem.**

Le directeur est au courant d'un service spécial qu'il doit me rendre à cause d'un problème médical.

■ **Does anyone here speak English?**

Y a-t-il quelqu'un ici qui parle anglais?

■ **I/she/he must follow a special diet because of diabetes.**

Je/elle/il dois suivre un régime spécial à cause du diabète.

■ **All food and drink must be completely free of sugar or sweetening.**

Tout—nourritures, boissons—doit être absolument sans sucre ou substance pour sucrer.

■ **Everything must be prepared without the ingredients on this list.**

Aucun des ingrédients de cette liste ne doivent figurer dans ce que je peux manger.

■ **A mistake can cause serious illness.**

Une erreur peut avoir des conséquences graves.

- **Does this dish contain any of the sweeteners on this list?**
Est-ce que ce plat contient un ou plusieurs de ces sucres sur la liste?

- **Can you prepare this dish/juice/beverage without sweetening?**
Pouvez-vous préparer ce plat/ce jus/cette boisson sans sucre ou substance pour sucrer?

- **Are the fruits/vegetables in this dish fresh/canned/frozen?**
Les fruits/les légumes de ce plat sont-ils frais/en conserve ou surgelés?

- **If it is canned or frozen in syrup, please drain all the liquid.**
Si c'est d'une boîte de conserve ou surgelé dans du sirop, s'il vous plaît, égouttez-le complètement.

- **Do you have any artificial sweetener?**
Avez-vous du sucre artificiel — une imitation de sucre?

- **If you are not sure, please tell me/ask the chef/the maitre d'.**
Si vous n'êtes pas sûr, s'il vous plaît dites-le-moi/demandez au chef ou au maître d'hôtel.

- **I would like to speak to the chef/to the maitre d'.**
Je voudrais parler au chef/au maître d'hôtel.

- **Do you have a microwave oven/a pressure cooker?**
Auriez-vous un four à micro-ondes/une marmite à pression?

(If the answer is *yes*, then ask:)

- **Can you prepare a single portion of _____, plain/without seasoning/gravy/sauce/sugar/butter/fat/oil?**
Pouvez-vous préparer une portion de _____ très simple/sans assaisonnement/jus/sauce/sucre/beurre/gras/huile?

■ **A mistake has been made. This is not what I ordered.**
Il y a une erreur. Ce n'est pas ce que j'ai commandé.

# The Low-Fat and Low-Cholesterol Diet

The following list of "not permitted" items may vary from the foods your physician has instructed you to avoid. To make the list easier for others to read, cross out the items that do not apply to you, and write in, PRINTING LEGIBLY, things you must avoid. Select them from the food lists on pages 175–194.

To make sure your food and drinks are prepared properly, consult *Appendix 3: French Food Preparation.* Use it together with other appropriate pages when ordering meals.

Some good news for meat lovers: French cuts of meat are on the lean side and the well-marbled steak is a rarity. Fat is carefully trimmed from meat in restaurants and butcher shops. However, since there are exceptions to every rule, we've included a request in your scenario for well-trimmed meat.

The easiest way to keep your fat intake low is to avoid gravies and sauces. Order dishes like broiled or baked fish that can be prepared quickly and without butter or sauce. A grilled steak served without butter, gravy or sauce is also a good choice. Breast of chicken can be very lean and greaseless too. But don't forget to have the skin removed; that's where most of the fat is concentrated. The light meat of chicken is leaner than the dark meat. How do you ask for the light meat of chicken? *"J'aimerais le blanc de poulet."* (I would like the light meat of chicken.) And don't forget to preface this and all other special requests with *s'il vous plaît* (please). It helps, particularly when a restaurant is crowded and its staff pushed.

More good news: low-fat yogurt is growing in popularity. In fact, you'll find magazine advertisements for completely fat-free yogurt. It's in the supermarkets, and you may also find it in some restaurants. If you want a low-fat yogurt, ask: *"Avez-vous du yoghurt maigre?"* (Do you have low-fat yogurt?)

# Foods Not Permitted — Aliments Interdits

- all animal fats—gras animal
- all fats—tous les gras
- all oils—toutes les huiles
- avocado—avocat
- bacon fat—saindoux, bacon
- butter—beurre
- canned meat/fish—viande/poisson en conserve
- cheese sauces—sauces au fromage
- chocolate—chocolat
- cocoa—cacao
- cocoa butter—beurre de noix de coco
- coconut—noix de coco
- coconut oil—huile de noix de coco ou copra
- cold cuts—charcuterie
- cream—crème fraîche
- eggs—oeufs
- egg yolk—jaune d'oeuf
- fried foods—fritures
- gravy—jus
- ground meat—viande hachée
- hydrogenated oil—huile hydrogénée
- kidney—rognon

- lard—saindoux
- liver—foie
- margarine—margarine
- mayonnaise—mayonnaise
- nuts—noix
- olive oil—huile d'olive
- organ meats—abats
- palm kernel oil—huile de palmiste
- palm oil—huile de palme
- part skim milk—lait ½ écrèmé
- peanut oil—huile d'arachide
- salad dressing (oil)—vinaigrette
- sauce—sauce
- sausage—saucisse
- shortening—gras
- shrimp—crevettes
- sour cream—crème aigre
- whole milk—lait complet
- yogurt/cheese made with whole or part skim milk—yoghourt/fromage fait au lait entier ou écrèmé

# The Low-Fat and Low-Cholesterol Scenario

If you can't pronounce the French, point to the appropriate phrases. For some sample replies to your questions, turn to *Appendix 3: French Food Preparation* and show it to your respondent.

- **I have a reservation. My name is _____.**
  J'ai réservé. Je m'appelle _____.

- **Please tell the manager I am here.**
  S'il vous plaît, dites au directeur que je suis ici.

- **The manager knows about the special service I need because of a medical problem.**
  Le directeur est au courant d'un service spécial qu'il doit me rendre à cause d'un problème médical.

- **Does anyone here speak English?**
  Y a-t-il quelqu'un ici qui parle anglais?

- **I/she/he must follow a special diet because of a serious medical problem.**
  Je/elle/il dois suivre un régime spécial à cause d'un problème médical très sérieux.

- **All food and drink must be fat-free.**
  Tous les plats et boissons doivent être préparés sans gras.

- **Everything must be prepared without the ingredients on this list.**
  Aucun des produits ou ingrédients de cette liste ne doivent figurer dans la préparation des plats que je peux manger.

- **Nothing can be fried.**
  Rien ne peut être frit.

- **All visible fat must be trimmed before cooking.**
  Tout le gras visible doit être retiré avant la cuisson.

- **A mistake can cause serious illness.**
  Une erreur peut avoir des conséquences graves.

207

■ **Does this dish contain any _____?**
Ce plat contient-il _____?

■ **Can you prepare this dish without _____?**
Pouvez-vous préparer ce plat sans _____?

■ **Can you prepare this dish with _____ instead of _____?**
Pouvez-vous préparer ce plat avec _____ au lieu de _____?

■ **Does this dish contain anything on this list?**
Ce plat contient-il un ou plusieurs des ingrédients de cette liste?

■ **Can you prepare this dish without any of the items on this list?**
Pouvez-vous préparer ce plat sans aucun des produits de cette liste?

■ **Are there any dishes on your menu that do not contain ingredients forbidden to me?**
Y a-t-il sur votre menu un plat qui ne contienne aucun des produits qui me sont interdits?

■ **Can you fry/prepare this dish with any of these oils: sunflower/corn/soy?**
Pouvez-vous faire frire/préparer ce plat avec une de ces huiles: huile de tournesol/maïs/soja?

■ **Please serve this plain, without any sauce/gravy.**
S'il vous plaît, servez ceci sans garniture, ni sauce, ni jus.

■ **If you are not sure, please tell me/ask the chef/the maître d'.**
Si vous n'êtes pas sûr, s'il vous plaît dites-le-moi/demandez au chef ou au maître d'hôtel.

- **I would like to speak to the chef/the maitre d'.**
  Je voudrais parler au chef/au maître d'hôtel.

- **Do you have a microwave oven/a pressure cooker?**
  Auriez-vous un four à micro-ondes/une marmite à pression?

  (If the answer is *yes*, then ask:)

- **Can you prepare a single portion of _____, plain/without seasoning/gravy/sauce/butter/oil/fats?**
  Pouvez-vous préparer une portion de _____, très simple/sans assaisonnement/jus/sauce/beurre/huile/gras?

- **A mistake has been made. This is not what I ordered.**
  Il y a une erreur. Ce n'est pas ce que j'ai commandé.

# The Ulcer, Bland, Soft, and Low-Residue Diet

The items on the following list of "not permitted" foods may vary from those your physician has instructed you to avoid. To make the list easier for others to read, cross out the items that do not apply to you, and add, PRINTING LEGIBLY, the things you cannot have. Select them from the food lists on pages 175–194.

To make sure your food and drink are prepared properly, consult *Appendix 3: French Food Preparation*. Use it together with other appropriate pages when ordering meals.

## Foods Not Permitted — Aliments Interdits

- bran—son
- catsup—ketchup
- clams—palourdes
- coconut—noix de coco
- corn—maïs
- dried fruits—fruits secs

*(continued on next page)*

## Foods Not Permitted—
## Aliments Interdits (continued)

- dried legumes—légumes secs
- fat—gras
- foods prepared with wine or liqueurs—mets préparés avec du vin ou de l'alcool
- fried foods—friture
- garlic—aïl
- gherkins—cornichons
- gravy—jus
- herbs—herbes aromatiques
- horseradish—raiford
- lard—saindoux
- meat broth—consommé de viande
- mustard—moutarde
- nuts/seeds—noix/graines
- olives—olives
- onions—oignons
- oysters—huîtres
- paprika—paprika
- peas—petits pois
- pepper—poivre
- pickled meat/fish—viande/poisson en saumure
- pork—porc
- raisins—raisins secs
- rice—riz
- salt—sel
- sauce—sauce
- seasoning—assaisonnement/aromate
- shallots—échalotes
- sharp (strong) cheese—fromage fort
- spices—épices
- vinegar—vinaigre
- wild rice—riz sauvage

# The Ulcer, Bland, Soft, and Low-Residue Scenario

If you cannot pronounce the French, point to appropriate phrases. For some sample replies to your questions, turn to *Appendix 3: French Food Preparation* and show it to your respondent.

**■ I have a reservation. My name is _____.**

J'ai réservé. Je m'appelle _____.

**■ Please tell the manager I am here.**

S'il vous plaît, dites au directeur que je suis ici.

**■ The manager knows about the special service I need because of a medical problem.**

Le directeur est au courant d'un service spécial qu'il doit me rendre à cause d'un problème médical.

- **Does anyone here speak English?**
Y a-t-il quelqu'un ici qui parle anglais?

- **I/she/he must follow a special diet for a stomach problem.**
Je/elle/il doit suivre un régime spécial à cause d'une maladie d'estomac.

- **Everything must be prepared without spices/seasoning.**
Tout doit être préparé sans épices/assaisonnement/aromates.

- **Nothing can be fried. Food must be baked/broiled/stewed/poached.**
Rien ne peut être frit. La nourriture doit être cuite au four/à la grillade/à l'étuvée/pochée.

- **A mistake can cause serious illness.**
Une erreur peut avoir des conséquences graves.

- **Please bake/broil/stew/poach this dish.**
S'il vous plaît, faites ce plat au four/à la grillade/à l'étuvée/poché.

- **Can you bake/broil/stew/poach this dish?**
Pouvez-vous faire ce plat au four/en grillade/à l'étuvée/poché?

- **Everything must be prepared without the ingredients on this list. Please read it. Thank you.**
Tout doit être préparé sans un seul des ingrédients de cette liste. S'il vous plaît, lisez-la. Merci.

- **Does this dish contain any _____?**
Est-ce que ce plat contient _____?

- **Can you prepare this dish without _____?**
Pouvez-vous préparer ce plat sans _____?

■ **Can you prepare this dish with _____ instead of _____?**

Pouvez-vous préparer ce plat avec _____ au lieu de _____?

■ **If you are not sure, please tell me/ask the chef/the maitre d'.**

Si vous n'êtes pas sûr, s'il vous plaît dites-le-moi/demandez au chef/au maître d'hotel.

■ **Can you prepare something bland and simple like a platter of plain baked fish, steamed or plain boiled potatoes, tender carrots or spinach/green beans/without seasoning, without spices?**

Pouvez-vous préparer quelque chose de simple et de pas relevé, par exemple du poisson au four sans assaisonnement et des pommes vapeur ou des pommes à l'anglaise/des carottes/des épinards/des haricots verts sans aromates, sans épices?

■ **Do you have a microwave oven/a pressure cooker?**

Auriez-vous un four à micro-ondes/une marmite à pression?

(If the answer is *yes,* then ask:)

■ **Can you prepare a single portion of _____, plain/without seasoning/gravy/sauce?**

Pouvez-vous préparer une portion de _____, très simple/sans assaisonnement/jus/sauce?

■ **A mistake has been made. This is not what I ordered.**

Il y a une erreur. Ce n'est pas ce que j'ai commandé.

■ **I would like to speak to the chef/the maitre d'.**

Je voudrais parler au chef/au maître d'hôtel.

# Design Your Own Scenario for a Custom-made Diet

If, for health, personal or religious reasons, you require a special diet that does not appear in this repertoire, you can produce your own script. We've made it easy for you by supplying the phrases on the following pages. To fill in the blanks of phrases you plan to use, do the following:

**1.** On a separate sheet of paper, prepare a list of foods you cannot eat.

**2.** To translate them into French, use the "not permitted" lists under the other diets and the food lists on pages 175–194; you may also find the supplementary lists at the end of this chapter useful.

**3.** Copy the list into this book, PRINTING LEGIBLY in the spaces provided under the heading, "not permitted." PRINT it in French *and* English.

**4.** PRINT the French words, where applicable, in the blanks in the script.

**5.** Don't forget to use *Appendix 3: French Food Preparation* to explain how you want your food prepared.

| Foods Not Permitted | Aliments Interdits |
|---|---|
| _____ | _____ |
| _____ | _____ |
| _____ | _____ |
| _____ | _____ |
| _____ | _____ |
| _____ | _____ |
| _____ | _____ |
| _____ | _____ |
| _____ | _____ |
| _____ | _____ |
| _____ | _____ |
| _____ | _____ |

# The Custom-made Scenario

If you can't pronounce the French, point to the appropriate phrases. For some sample replies to your questions, turn to *Appendix 3: French Food Preparation* and show it to your respondent.

■ **I have a reservation. My name is _____.**
J'ai réservé. Je m'appelle _____.

■ **Please tell the manager I am here.**
S'il vous plaît, dites au directeur que je suis ici.

■ **The manager knows about the special service I need because of a medical problem.**
Le directeur est au courant d'un service spécial qu'il doit me rendre à cause d'un problème médical.

■ **The manager knows about the special diet I need.**
Le directeur est au courant du régime spécial dont j'ai besoin.

■ **Does anyone here speak English?**
Y a-t-il quelqu'un ici qui parle anglais?

■ **I/she/he must follow a special diet.**
Je/elle/il doit suivre un régime spécial.

■ **All food and drink must be completely free of _____.**
Tout—nourritures, boissons—doit être absolument sans _____.

■ **Everything must be prepared without the items on this list.**
Tout doit être préparé sans aucun des ingrédients de cette liste.

- **A mistake can cause serious illness.**
  Une erreur peut avoir des conséquences graves.

- **Does this dish contain any _____?**
  Ce plat contient-il _____?

- **Does this dish contain anything on this list?**
  Y a-t-il dans ce plat aucun des ingrédients de cette liste?

- **Can you prepare this dish without _____?**
  Pouvez-vous préparer ce plat sans _____?

- **Show me on the menu which dishes you can prepare without _____.**
  Montrez-moi sur le menu quels plats vous pouvez préparer sans _____.

- **Show me on the menu which dishes you can prepare without any of the items on this list.**
  Montrez-moi sur le menu quels plats vous pouvez préparer sans un seul des ingrédients de cette liste.

- **Are there any dishes on the menu that do not contain ingredients forbidden to me?**
  Y a-t-il des plats sur le menu qui ne contiennent aucun des ingrédients qui me sont interdits?

- **If you are not sure, please tell me/ask the chef/the maitre d'.**
  Si vous n'êtes pas sûr, s'il vous plaît, demandez au chef/au maître d'hôtel.

- **I would like to speak to the chef/the maitre d'.**
  Je voudrais parler au chef/au maître d'hôtel.

- **Can you prepare something simple for me in your kitchen that is appropriate for my diet? For example:** _____.
  Pouvez-vous me préparer quelque chose de simple qui serait approprié à mon régime? Par exemple: _____.

- **Do you have a microwave oven/a pressure cooker?**
  Avez-vous un four à micro-ondes/une marmite à pression?

  (If the answer is *yes*, then ask:)

- **Can you prepare a single portion of** _____ **without** _____?
  Pouvez-vous préparer une portion de _____ sans _____?

- **A mistake has been made. This is not what I ordered.**
  Il y a une erreur. Ce n'est pas ce que j'ai commandé.

To compose a list of forbidden items, consult the food lists on pages 175–194, the collection of no-nos for the other scenarios, and this sampling of foods that may cause reactions in some allergenic and otherwise sensitive individuals.

# Possible Forbidden Items – Aliments Interdits

- barley—orge
- barley cereal—céréale d'orge
- barley flour—farine d'orge
- beef—boeuf
- beets—betteraves
- bran—son
- buckwheat—sarrasin (blé noir)
- buckwheat cereal—céréale de sarrasin (blé noir)
- buckwheat flour—farine de sarrasin (blé noir)
- cane sugar—sucre de cane
- chocolate—chocolat
- cinnamon—cannelle
- citrus fruits—agrumes
- coconut—noix de coco
- coffee—café
- cola—cola
- corn—maïs

- corn products—produits contenant du maïs
- dates—dattes
- eggs—oeufs
- figs—figues
- fish—poisson
- legumes—légumes secs
- lettuce—laitue
- malt—malt, orge germé
- milk—lait
- nuts—noix
- oat flour—farine d'avoine
- oatmeal bread—pain aux flocons d'avoine
- oatmeal cereal—céréale aux flocons d'avoine
- oatmeal stuffing—farce contenant des flocons d'avoine
- oats—avoine
- peanuts—cacahuètes, arachides
- pork—porc
- potato—pomme de terre
- rice—riz
- ripe beans—haricots écossés
- rye—seigle
- rye bread—pain de seigle
- rye bread crumbs—miettes de pain de seigle
- rye cereal—céréale de seigle
- rye flour—farine de seigle
- shellfish—coquillages
- soybeans—soja
- string beans—haricots verts
- tomato—tomate
- wheat—blé
- wheat bread—pain à la farine de blé
- wheat cereal—céréale au blé
- wheat crumbs—chapelure
- wheat flour—farine de blé
- wheat germ—germe de blé
- wheat germ oil—huile de germe de blé
- wheat stuffing—farce contenant du blé (ou du pain)
- yeast—levure

# Medical Aid

Read these pages now. They will make things easier for you later.

In an acute emergency ask a French-speaking person to telephone for help for you. You will find the phrase for such a request under *Emergencies.* Memorize it now.

## U.S. Embassy and Consular Assistance in France

If you are visiting Paris, you can obtain a list of qualified English-speaking physicians from the American Embassy. It's a good thing to keep handy. But why wait for an emergency? Get your umbrella before it rains by dropping in for your list at the:

**Embassy of the United States** — 2 Avenue Gabriel, Paris. Telephone: area code (01) 296-1202 or 261-8075.

Similar consular services are available in other French cities, too:

**Bordeaux** — 4, Rue Esprit des Lois. Telephone: area code (56) 52 65 95.

**Lyon** — 7, Quai Général Sarrail. Telephone: area code (78) 24 68 49.

**Marseille** — 9, Rue Armeny. Telephone: area code (91) 54 92 00.

**Strasbourg** — 15, Avenue d'Alsace. Telephone: area code (88) 35 31/04/ or /05/06/.

# Emergencies

■ **Help!**
   Au secours!

- **Police!**
  Police!

- **Fire!**
  Au feu!

- **I am ill.**
  Je suis malade.

- **She is ill.**
  Elle est malade.

- **He is ill.**
  Il est malade.

- **Call a doctor right away.**
  Appelez un médecin immédiatement.

- **Call an ambulance right away.**
  Appelez une ambulance immédiatement.

- **Take me/us to a doctor right away.**
  Emmenez-moi/nous chez un médecin immédiatement.

- **Take me/us to a hospital right away.**
  Emmenez-moi/nous à un hôpital immédiatement.

- **Is there a doctor in the building?**
  Y a-t-il un médecin dans cette maison?

- **I cannot speak French. Please call this number for me.**
  Je ne peux pas parler français. S'il vous plaît, appelez-
  moi ce n° de téléphone.

# Emergency Telephone Numbers

When you check in at your lodgings, ask the desk clerk or manager for emergency numbers. Sure, you'll feel funny making such a request before you've even seen your room or unpacked your bags, but it's worth the discomfort. Practice these phrases, and when you get the numbers, put them in the blanks of the *Emergency Telephone Numbers* box below. Or better yet, ask the clerk to write them in for you. If you show him or her the book with this official-looking box, your request won't appear quite so strange.

■ **Emergency numbers belong in this box. Would you mind filling it in for me? Thank you.**
Il me faut les numéros à appeler en cas d'urgence. Cela vous ennuierait-il de me les écrire? Merci.

---

**Emergency Telephone Numbers**

En cas d'urgence, appelez ces n° de téléphone.

Ambulance—Ambulance: _____

Fire—(Feu) Pompiers: _____

Police—Police: _____

---

# Asking for Help

■ **Where is the nearest doctor?**
Où se trouve le médecin le plus proche?

- **Where is the nearest hospital/clinic?**
  Où se trouve l'hôpital/la clinique la plus proche?

- **Where is the nearest first-aid station?**
  Où se trouve le poste de secours le plus proche?

- **Where is the nearest pharmacy?**
  Où se trouve la pharmacie la plus proche?

- **Where is the nearest English-speaking doctor?**
  Où puis-je trouver un médecin qui parle anglais?

- **Is there an English-speaking doctor here?**
  Y a-t-il ici un médecin qui parle anglais?

- **Is there a hospital here with English-speaking doctors?**
  Y a-t-il ici un hôpital avec des médecins qui parlent anglais?

- **At what time can the doctor come?**
  A quelle heure le médecin pourrait-il venir?

- **What are the office hours?**
  A quelles heures sont les consultations?

- **Please PRINT the information. Thank you.**
  S'il vous plaît, écrivez ce renseignement en caractères D'IMPRIMERIE. Merci beaucoup.

- **What is the doctor's name, address, and telephone number?**
  Quel est le nom, l'adresse, et le n° de téléphone du médecin?

- **Please show me where it is on this map.**
  S'il vous plaît, montrez-moi sur cette carte où cela se trouve.

- **Please show me on the map where we are now.**
S'il vous plaît, montrez-moi sur cette carte où nous nous trouvons.

- **Please draw a map/sketch for me.**
S'il vous plaît, faites-moi un dessin.

- **I cannot speak French. Please phone for me.**
Je ne peux pas parler français. S'il vous plaît, télé-phonez pour moi.

- **Does anyone here speak English?**
Y a-t-il quelqu'un ici qui parle anglais?

- **I need an interpreter.**
Il me faut un interprète.

# Numbers

0 — zéro
1 — un, une
2 — deux
3 — trois
4 — quatre
5 — cinq
6 — six
7 — sept
8 — huit
9 — neuf
10 — dix
11 — onze
12 — douze
13 — treize
14 — quatorze
15 — quinze
16 — seize
17 — dix-sept
18 — dix-huit
19 — dix-neuf
20 — vingt
21 — vingt et un

22 — vingt-deux
30 — trente
31 — trente et un
32 — trente-deux
40 — quarante
41 — quarante et un
42 — quarante-deux
50 — cinquante
60 — soixante
70 — soixante-dix
80 — quatre-vingts
90 — quatre-vingt-dix
100 — cent
101 — cent un
200 — deux cents
250 — deux cent cinquante
300 — trois cents
500 — cinq cents
1000 — mille
half — demi or moitié
quarter — quart

# Section Five:
# Say It
# in Italian

# Italian Pronunciation

Like Spanish, Italian is a phonetic language; that is, the spoken word closely matches its spelling. As a result, pronunciation of Italian is relatively easy. Unlike English, Italian vowels are always pronounced clearly and are the same whether they occur in a stressed or unstressed position. There are, however, two variants for **E** and **O**.

## Vowels

**A**   as in **A**LWAYS, **A**RMY
**E**   as in TH**E**Y without final /i/ glide, or as in B**E**T
**I**   as in MACH**I**NE
**O**   as in B**A**LD, B**A**LL, or sometimes as in L**O**W, without final /u/ glide
**U**   as in R**U**LE

## Consonants

In Italian, a double consonant is pronounced with more force, and/or is held longer than the single consonant sound. A single consonant lengthens a preceding stressed vowel, while a double consonant shortens a preceding stressed vowel.

**C**     before A, O, U like **K**ITE: *carne*
**C**     before E, I like **CH**EST: *cento*
**CH**    before E, I like **K**ITE: *chilo*
**CI**    before A, O, U like **CH**EST: *ciurma*
**G**     before A, O, U like **G**O: *gambero*
**G**     before E, I like **G**EM: *gentile*
**GH**    before E, I like **G**O: *ghermire*
**GI**    before A, O, U like **G**EM (**J**OHN): *giorno*
**GLI**   like **LL** in MI**LL**ION: *aglio, gli*
**GN**    like **NY** in CA**NY**ON: *ogni*

| H   | is silent: *ha* |
| --- | --- |
| QU  | like **QU**EST: *questo* |
| S   | when before B, D, G, L, M, N, R, V like **S** in RO**S**E |
| SC  | before A, O, U like **SK** in A**SK**: *pesca* |
| SC  | before E, I like **SH** in FI**SH**: *mescere* |
| SCH | before E, I like **SK** in A**SK**: *pesche* |
| Z   | is sometimes voiceless, as in BE**TS**: *marzo;* sometimes voiced, as in BE**DS**: *orzo* |

# Inflection

Italian words are usually accented on the second-to-the-last syllable: *andare* is *an-DA-re; mandare, man-DA-re; carne, CAR-ne; spaghetti, spa-GHET-ti;* and *formaggio, for-MAG-gio.* Occasionally, it falls on the third to the last: *telefono* is *te-LE-fo-no.* Printed accent marks are not used except when the stress falls on the last syllable: *caffè* is *caf-FÈ; città* is *cit-TÀ.*

# Basic Expressions in Italian

- **Yes**
  Sí

- **No**
  No

- **Please**
  Per favore

- **Thank you**
  Grazie

- **Excuse me**
  Mi scusi

- **Pardon me**
  Mi scusi

- **Good morning or Good afternoon/Good evening**
  Buon giorno/Buona sera

- **Good night/Good-bye**
  Buona notte/ArrivederLa, Arrivederci (informal)

- **Where is the ladies'/men's room?**
  Dov'è la toilette per signore/per uomini?

- **My name is _____.**
  Mi chiamo _____.

- **I am staying at _____.**
  Sto presso _____.

- **Can you help me?**
  Mi puó aiutare?

- **Do you speak English?**
  Parla inglese?

- **Does anyone here speak English?**
  C'è qualcuno qui che parla inglese?

- **Can you find anyone who speaks English?**
  Puó trovare qualcuno che parla inglese?

- **I do not understand.**
  Non capisco.

- **Please speak slowly.**
  Per favore, parli piú piano.

- **Please repeat it.**
  Ripeta, per favore.

- **Please PRINT the directions.**
  Per favore, scriva IN STAMPATELLO le istruzioni.

- **Please PRINT it.**
  Per favore, lo scriva IN STAMPATELLO.

- **Please PRINT the name, address, and telephone number.**
  Per favore, scriva IN STAMPATELLO il nome, l'indirizzo e il numero di telefono.

- **Please show me on this map.**
  Per favore, me lo indichi su questa cartina.

■ **Please show me on this map where I am.**
Per favore, mi indichi dove sono su questa cartina.

■ **Please draw a map/sketch for me.**
Per favore, mi disegni una cartina. Mi faccia un disegnino.

■ **Please call this number for me. Thank you.**
Per favore, mi chiami questo numero. Grazie.

■ **Where is the nearest _____?**
Dov'è il piú vicino _____?

   ■ **hospital/clinic**
   ospedale/la clinica

   ■ **first aid facility**
   pronto soccorso

   ■ **diet/health food/natural food restaurant**
   ristorante di macrobiotica/cibi organici/cibi naturali

■ **Is the restaurant open/closed now?**
È aperto/chiuso ora il ristorante?

■ **Please point to the days and hours it is open/closed.**
Per favore, mi indichi i giorni di esercizio e l'orario del ristorante.

■ **Monday**
lunedí

■ **Tuesday**
martedí

■ **Wednesday**
mercoledí

- **Thursday**
  giovedí

- **Friday**
  venerdí

- **Saturday**
  sabato

- **Sunday**
  domenica

- **a quarter past**
  e un quarto

- **half past**
  e mezzo

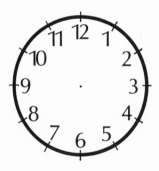

- **a quarter to**
  meno un quarto

- **noon**
  mezzogiorno

- **midnight**
  mezzanotte

- **in the morning/afternoon/evening/night**
  di mattina/di pomeriggio/di sera/di notte

- **How much is this? Please write it down. (For a list of numbers, see page 285.)**
  Quanto costa? Per favore, me lo scriva.

- **Do you have _____?**
  Ha _____?

- **I would like _____.**
  Vorrei _____.

- **Please give me _____.**
  Per favore, mi dia _____.

# Dining Out in Italy

This section is divided into three parts. Part 1 includes a description of the hours for mealtimes, the available types of eating establishments, cover charges and tipping customs, plus some techniques of finding a restaurant and making reservations. Also, after finding a restaurant, there are questions included which you may need to ask, such as how to find a smoke-free spot. Part 2 gives some basic food lists arranged in breakfast, lunch, and dinner order. Part 3 contains a series of diet scenarios, each linked to specific health problems plus a scenario adaptable to the needs of travelers on special diets not covered in the more specific scenarios. Look them over now and check those items that will come in handy later.

## Part 1

### Mealtimes in Italy

Breakfast is served only in eating establishments attached to hotels. Their hours can vary, so inquire at your hotel. Italian breakfasts usually consist of coffee with milk (*caffelatte*), espresso plus steamed milk (*cappuccino*) or cocoa, served with rolls, butter and jam, or pastries. Italians often have their breakfasts at a *caffè* or *bar* where such items are also served. Lunch is usually the main Italian meal. Dinner is eaten late, and it is not uncommon to find restaurants serving after 10:00 P.M.

Breakfast:  served between 7:00 and 10:00
Lunch:  served between 12:00 and 2:00
Dinner:  served between 7:30 or 8:00 and 10:00

# Types of Eating Establishments in Italy

*Albergo* — a hotel; almost all *alberghi* have restaurants.

*Bar/Caffè* — alcoholic beverages, coffee, ice cream, pastry, and sometimes simple sandwiches. Popular place for an Italian-style breakfast.

*Girarrosto* — features meats cooked on a spit in electric ovens or over coals. Some may have cafeteria-style food as well.

*Hotel* — menus can be simple or extensive, depending on the class of the hotel. Prices vary accordingly.

*Locanda* — an inn, generally in a rural area or the mountains. Usually equipped with a kitchen that turns out tasty, home-cooked meals.

*Osteria* — a smaller bar-restaurant; unpretentious, usually frequented by locals. Clientele ranges from would-be chic in search of genuine cooking to working class. Food can be excellent, although menus are not usually extensive.

*Pizzeria* — serves pizzas and fried dough specialties; beer or cola, sometimes wine offered.

*Ristorante* — a restaurant's class determines its prices and menu.

*Rosticceria* — generally serves roast chicken (plus other roast specialties), and deli or cafeteria-style foods like salads and sandwiches. Foods can usually be taken out.

*Taverna* — a smaller drinking and/or eating establishment, rustic and unpretentious; like an *osteria,* it caters to locals, though nowadays it may simply be a restaurant with rustic decor.

*Tavola Calda* — much like a cafeteria; prepared dishes, sandwiches, and salads for quick lunches.

*Trattoria* — a smaller restaurant, unpretentious, and rustic in atmosphere featuring home cooking. In the same class as the *osteria.*

*Vini e Cucina* — as the name implies, local wines in quantity and a simple kitchen with unpretentious home cooking. Generally caters to the working class, but food can be tasty—if not excellent—and inexpensive. Only for veteran travelers!

# Tipping and Cover Charges in Italy

Usually, the food bill (*il conto*) will include a charge for service (*servizio*), which varies from 10 to 15 percent of the total. An additional tip, however, is customarily left on the table for the waiter. How much is up to the customer and depends on the size of the original service charge and the quality of the service itself. Three to 5 percent is average.

Almost all eating establishments have a cover charge (*pane e coperto*) to pay for bread and linens. This is usually specified on menus and varies, according to the class of the restaurant, between 50¢ and $1.00.

# A Piacere — to Your Taste . . .

These words occasionally appear on Italian menus, and they are an invitation to you to order dishes tailored to your taste at a specified charge. If a blank space appears after these tempting words and no price is quoted, beware. The maitre d' is then free to set his own price, something that he feels is fair for the service rendered.

# Making Reservations in Italian Restaurants

Let the chef know you're coming and that you must observe a special diet. Ask your hotel manager or desk clerk to phone the restaurant for you. If you don't speak Italian, and they don't speak English, simply point to the appropriate phrases.

Ask the desk clerk or hotel manager to read the following section before he or she phones for a reservation. To describe your needs, fill in the blanks with words and phrases selected from the "not permitted" list under your diet, the diet's scenario, the food lists, and the food preparation information in *Appendix 4.*

- **Can you recommend a good, but not too expensive restaurant?**

Mi può consigliare un ristorante buono ma che non sia troppo caro?

- **I have/she/he has a special problem and would like you to read the following:**

Ho/ha un problema medico, e vorrei che leggesse cosa seque:

- **I must ask a favor of you. I have/she/he has a medical problem and must observe a very special diet.**

Le vorrei chiedere di farmi una cortesia. Ho/ha un problema medico e devo/deve osservare una dieta speciale.

- **Since I cannot speak Italian, may I ask you to phone the restaurant for me and explain the problem?**

Perché non so parlare italiano, mi farebbe la cortesia di telefonare al ristorante e spiegare il problema?

- **May I ask you to do a favor for me/for us? Please phone this restaurant and make a reservation for me for a party of _____ for lunch/dinner. For today/tomorrow. For Monday/ Tuesday/Wednesday/Thursday/Friday/Saturday/Sunday. At _____ o'clock.**

Mi/ci può fare una cortesia? Per favore, chiami questo ristorante e faccia una prenotazione per me/ per _____ persone per colazione/per cena. Per oggi/domani. Per lunedí/martedí/mercoledí/giovedí/ venerdí/sabato/domenica. A _____.

- **I/she/he cannot eat anything containing _____.**

Non posso/può mangiare niente che contenga

_____.

- **A mistake can cause serious illness.**

Un errore può provocare una grave malattia.

- **Ask the maitre d' if he will be so kind as to arrange for simple substitutions in the dishes served to me.**

  Domandi al maitre d'hotel se potrebbe essere cosí gentile da provvedere che nei miei piatti vengano eseguite delle semplici sostituzioni.

- **For example, for lunch/dinner I would like _____ or _____.**

  Per esempio, per cena/per pranzo vorrei _____ oppure _____.

- **It should be _____ (method of preparation—see *Appendix 4*).**

  Dovrebbe essere _____.

- **It should not contain any _____.**

  Non dovrebbe contenere _____.

- **Please ask for the name of the person with whom you are speaking. Write it down (PRINT it) for me. Thank you very much.**

  Per favore, chieda il nome della persona con cui sto parlando. Me lo scriva IN STAMPATELLO. Grazie mille.

- **Please PRINT the name, address, and telephone number. Thank you.**

  Per favore, scriva IN STAMPATELLO il nome, l'indirizzo, e il numero di telefono. Grazie.

After the call has been made, you can ask:

- **Have you made the reservation?**

  Ha fatto la prenotazione?

- **Did they understand my/her/his problem?**

  Hanno capito il mio/il suo problema?

**Are they willing to arrange for special dishes?**
Sono disposti a preparare piatti speciali?

You'll find these phrases helpful if you choose a restaurant on the spur of the moment.

**Are reservations necessary?**
È necessario fare una prenotazione?

**A table for _____, please. (See list of numbers on page 285.)**
Un tavolo per _____, per favore.

**Do you have a nonsmoking section?**
Ha una sezione per non-fumatori?

**Please, can you seat me/us as far away from smokers as possible?**
Per favore, mi/ci può far sedere il più lontano possibile dai fumatori?

**I have/she/he has a serious allergy to smoke.**
Ho/ha/una grave allergia al fumo.

**Where is the ladies'/men's room?**
Dov'è la toilette?

**Do you have _____?**
Ha _____?

**I would like _____.**
Vorrei _____.

- **Please give me _____.**
  Per favore, mi dia _____.
    - **glass of water (See pages 26–27 about water.)**
      un bicchiere d'acqua.
    - **bottle of plain water sealed/unopened**
      una bottiglia di acqua semplice chiusa/aperta
    - **bottle of carbonated water unopened**
      una bottiglia di acqua gassata aperta
    - **bottle of mineral water unopened**
      una bottiglia di acqua minerale/aperta
    - **fork/knife/spoon/napkin/straws**
      una forchetta/un coltello/un cucchiaio/un tovagliolo/cannucce

# Fish and Shellfish in Italy: A Word of Caution

Be sure any fish or shellfish you eat is well cooked. Mediterranean waters have not been given a clean bill of health, and it's best to avoid shellfish taken from them. Shellfish from northern waters are okay.

# Part 2

The phrases and food lists in this section will be a big help in restaurants, supermarkets, and food stores. For a list of numbers to interpret bills, see page 285.

# Breakfast

Most hotels in Italy serve a continental breakfast consisting of fresh rolls, butter, jam, and coffee, tea, or hot chocolate. If your hotel has a restaurant, it may be possible to request something more like home but expect to pay extra for it, since a continental breakfast is usually included in the price of a night's lodging. Of course, if you are staying at a hotel that caters predominantly to American tourists or breakfasting in a large restaurant, you may not be limited to a roll and a beverage.

Breakfast is an important meal, especially if you plan to be active in the hours before lunchtime. A hearty breakfast will stave off the hunger that may trap you into stuffing yourself at lunch or dinner. So, if you want something more substantial than the traditional Italian breakfast, speak with the hotel manager or maitre d' the day or evening before your first morning meal. Try these phrases:

- **May I ask a special favor of you?**
  Le posso chiedere di farmi una cortesia?

- **Would it be possible to have _____ for breakfast?**
  Sarebbe possibile avere _____ a colazione?

Then select something from the lists of breakfast foods on the following pages, but keep it simple. If necessary, show your WALLET CARD; it will lend authority to a special request. If your food must be prepared in a special way, point to the appropriate phrases (*Appendix 4*). Better still, put it all down on paper before you approach the maitre d'. PRINT IT! Of course, you'll feel a little silly the very first time you make a special request and flash your WALLET CARD. Who wouldn't? But keep in mind that the hotel staff is anxious to make your stay a comfortable one. The important thing is to be polite and friendly when asking for a custom-made meal. After you've tried it once, you'll become an old hand at it.

# Fruit Juice – Succo di Frutta

Let's start with fruit juice. Orange juice is usually freshly squeezed in Italy. Other juices may be prepared from concentrate or frozen juice, and you may want to ask:

- **Is this juice prepared from concentrate/from frozen juice?**
  Questo succo di frutta è preparato da concentrato/ congelato?

- **I want only freshly squeezed/canned/bottled juice.**
  Voglio solamente spremute fresche/succo in scatola/bottiglia.

- **Do you have _____?**
  Ha _____?

- **I would like _____.**
  Vorrei _____.

- **Please give me _____.**
  Per favore, mi dia _____.

Select a fruit juice and ask for *succo di* (or *d'*) _____ (the juice of _____).

# Fruit Juices

*English—Italian*
- apple—mela
- apricot—albicocca
- grape—uva
- grapefruit—pompelmo
- lemon—limone
- lime—cedro
- orange—arancia
- peach—pesca
- pear—pera
- pineapple—ananas
- prune—prugna
- tomato—pomodoro

*Italian—English*
- albicocca—apricot
- ananas—pineapple
- arancia—orange
- cedro—lime
- limone—lemon
- mela—apple
- pera—pear
- pesca—peach
- pomodoro—tomato
- pompelmo—grapefruit
- prugna—prune
- uva—grape

# Fruit—Frutta

*English—Italian*
- apple—mela
- apricots—albicocche
- avocado—avocado
- banana—banana

*Italian—English*
- albicocche—apricots
- ananas—pineapple
- anguria—watermelon
- arancia—orange

*(continued on next page)*

**Dining Out**

**Italian**

# Fruit — Frutta (continued)

*English — Italian*

- blackberries — more
- cherries — ciliege
- coconut — cocco
- dates — datteri
- figs — fichi
- filberts — nocciole
- grapefruit — pompelmo
- grapes — uva
- lemon — limone
- lime — cedro
- medlars — nespole
- melon — melone
- mulberries — gelsi
- nectarines — percoche
- olives — olive
- orange — arancia
- peach — pesca
- pear — pera
- persimmon — cachi
- pineapple — ananas
- plums — susine/prugne
- pomegranate — melograno
- prickly pears — fichi d'India
- prunes — prugne
- raisins — uva passa
- raspberries — lamponi
- strawberries — fragole
- tangerine — mandarino
- walnuts — noci
- watermelon — anguria/cocomero

*Italian — English*

- avocado — avocado
- banana — banana
- cachi — persimmon
- cedro — lime
- ciliege — cherries
- cocco — coconut
- cocomero — watermelon
- datteri — dates
- fichi — figs
- fichi d'India — prickly pears
- fragole — strawberries
- gelsi — mulberries
- lamponi — raspberries
- limone — lemon
- mandarino — tangerine
- mela — apple
- melograno — pomegranate
- melone — melon
- more — blackberries
- nespole — medlars
- nocciole — filberts
- noci — walnuts
- olive — olives
- pera — pear
- percoche — nectarines
- pesca — peach
- pompelmo — grapefruit
- prugne — prunes/plums
- susine — plums
- uva — grapes
- uva passa — raisins

# Cereals – Cereali

Even though cereal is not a part of the breakfast menu in Italy, you may find it at a hotel that caters mainly to American tourists. You may want to ask before you order cereal:

■ **Please, would you check the label on the container and tell me if it contains salt/sodium/sugar/sweetener?**
Volete controllare l'etichetta del contenitore e assicurate se il contenitore contiene sale/sodio/zuccharo/dolcificante?

When ordering cold cereals at a hotel restaurant, you may ask:

■ **Do you have American boxed cereals?**
Ha cereali in scatola americani?

■ **Do you have corn flakes?**
Ha fiocchi di granturco?

## Hot Cereals

Before you order cooked cereal, you might want to give these instructions to the cook:

■ **Please cook it in unsalted water.**
Per favore, lo faccia cuocere senza sale.

■ **Don't put any _____ in it.**
Non ci metta _____.

■ **Please put some _____ in it.**
Per favore, ci metta _____.

Does your diet require a highly refined cereal, a baby cereal? If so, ask:

■ **Do you have any refined cereals suitable for babies?**
Ha cereali fini per neonati?

# Bread, Rolls, and Crackers — Pane, Panini, e Crackers

- rye—segale
- white—bianco
- whole wheat—integrale

■ **Please toast the bread.**
Per favore, vorrei pane tostato.

■ **Please warm the _____.**
Per favore, riscaldi _____.

You can try *pane condito* if you have a strong stomach. It's a bread laced with animal fats and bacon bits and very heavy! On the other hand, *panini all'olio,* rolls seasoned with olive oil, are very tasty and surprisingly light.

# Eggs — Uova

- fried—fritte
- hard-boiled—sode
- plain omelet—frittata
- poached—in camicia
- scrambled—strapazzate
- soft-boiled—alla coque

# Dairy Products — Latticini

Pasteurization of dairy products is routine in Italy. But if you are ordering milk, cheese or butter in a small village, you might want to ask:

■ **Is it pasteurized?**
È pastorizzato?

■ **Has it been refrigerated?**
È stato conservato in frigorifero?

- butter (usually unsalted)—burro
- butter, salted—burro salato
- diet (low-calorie) margarine—margarina dietetica
- main ingredient should be unhardened (liquid) vegetable oil—l'ingrediente principale dovrebbe essere olio vegetale non-idrogenato:
    - corn—olio di mais
    - olive—olio d'oliva
    - peanut—olio di arachidi
    - safflower—olio di cartamo
    - soy—olio di semi di soia
    - sunflower—olio di semi di girasole
- margarine (normally contains salt)—margarina
- margarine, salt-free—margarina senza sale

### Cheese—Formaggio

If you must know the fat content of a cheese you'd like to order, you could be in for trouble in Italy, because that information rarely appears on labels. What's worse, there is no Italian cheese with as low a fat content as American cottage cheese. Still, there are ways of finding relatively low-calorie cheeses, and we've included some phrases to guide you. When dining in a restaurant, you might ask:

■ **Is it made with whole milk?**
È fatto con latte intero?

■ **Is it made with skim milk?**
È fatto con latte scremato?

■ **Is it made with part skim milk?**
È fatto con latte parzialmente scremato?

■ **Has salt been added? (Even if salt has not been added, all cheeses have a high salt content!)**
C'è aggiunta di sale?

■ **Has cream been added?**
C'è aggiunta di panna?

■ **What percentage of fat does it contain?**
Qual è la percentuale di grassi?

■ **Please write it down. Thank you.**
Per favore, me lo scriva. Grazie.

■ **Do you have any low-fat/low-calorie/low-salt cheese?**
Ha formaggi a bassi livelli di grasso/con poche calorie/poco salati?

### Some Fresh Cheeses

There are several cheeses that are somewhat lower in fat than most of the cheeses you'll find in Italy. However, compared to low-fat cottage cheese or other diet cheeses, they still cannot be recommended to someone on a low-fat, low-cholesterol diet.

**Ricotta** — made from whole milk, either ewe or sheep's milk. Sheep's milk ricotta is delicious.

**Fior di Latte** — a type of mozzarella cheese; it's advertised in Italy as lower in fat and calories than most Italian cheeses.

**Mozzarella** — lower in salt and fat than most other cheeses. *Fior di latte* can be found everywhere in Italy, while *ricotta* and *mozzarella* tend to be more popular in the southern part of Italy (or from Rome on down).

### Yogurt—Yogurt

• low-fat yogurt—yogurt magro
■ **Is it made with skim milk?**
È fatto con latte scremato?

■ **Is it made with part skim milk?**
È fatto con latte parzialmente scremato?

### Cream—Panna

• nondairy creamer (almost unknown, but try anyway)— panna non latticina or sostituto artificale per latte
• sour cream—panna acida

### Milk—Latte

You won't find unhomogenized milk except in small villages, where most likely it will not be pasteurized either.
- buttermilk—siero di latte
- canned milk—latte in scatola
- condensed milk—latte condensato
- evaporated skim milk—latte evaporato scremato
- evaporated whole milk—latte evaporato intero
- fresh skim—fresco scremato
- fresh whole—fresco intero
- homogenized—omogenizzato
- pasteurized—pastorizzato
- powdered skim—scremato in polvere
- powdered whole—intero in polvere

# Spreads

What do you like on your bread, rolls or crackers?
- honey—miele
- jam—conserva di frutta
- jelly—gelatina di frutta
- marmalade—marmellata
- peanut butter (Peanut butter is hard to get at this time in Italy.)—pasta di arachidi

# Beverages—Bevande

Italians do not drink weak, American-style coffee. *Espresso* is their equivalent of "black coffee" and is often taken with sugar. *Caffelatte* is *Espresso* with a good bit of milk added. *Caffè macchiato* is coffee with a little milk or cream in it. *Cappuccino* is *Espresso* with frothy steamed milk injected into the coffee.

If you want decaffeinated coffee, ask for *caffè decaffeinato.*
- fruit juice—succo di frutta
- hot chocolate—cioccolata calda
- milk—latte

- tea—tè
- herb tea—infuso di erbe (*Camomilla*—camomile tea is popular.)

For an additional listing of beverages, see pages 256–257.

# Lunch and Dinner

Worried about preparation? Consult *Appendix 4: Italian Food Preparation.*

If you're on a restricted diet, you'll like meat in Italy. Beef is slaughtered young in this country and generally most of the fat is trimmed before cooking. Since Italians like their meat lean, American-style, marbled steaks are nonexistent. Nor is Italian meat aged as it is in the United States. Baby veal and veal are the most popular varieties. Italian veal is slaughtered very young and tends to be even younger than the American variety.

■ **What kind of meat is this?**

Che tipo di carne è questa?

■ **Please show me on this list.**

Per favore, me lo indichi su quest' elenco.

■ **I would like _____.**

Vorrei _____.
- chicken—pollo
- kid—capretto
- lamb—agnello
- lean·beef—manzo magro
- pork—maiale
- turkey—tacchino
- veal—vitello
    - baby veal—vitellino di latte

Here are some cuts of meat, listed by category—beef, lamb, pork, poultry, veal, and variety meats.

# Cuts of Meat

## English—Italian
### Beef—*Manzo/Bue*
- baby beef, very lean—vitellone magro
- beefsteak—bistecca
- chuck—spalla
- filet mignon—filetto
- flank steak—petto/falda
- liver (low in fat but high in cholesterol)—fegato
- roast beef—rosbif
- round (usually round roast, but you can have a slice cut off for steak)—girello
- rump—pezza/mela/scamone
- tripe (very popular)—trippa

### Lamb—*Agnello*
- leg—cosciotto
- loin chops—costolette
- loin roast—sella
- rib—costata
- shank—peduccio
- shoulder—spalla

### Pork—*Maiale*
- pork chops—braciole di maiale
- pork cutlets—cotolette di maiale
- suckling pig—porcellino di latte
- tenderloin (very lean, no fat, tender)—filetto di maiale

## Italian—English
### *Manzo/Bue*—Beef
- bistecca—beefsteak
- falda—flank steak
- fegato—liver
- filetto—filet mignon
- girello—usually round roast, but you can have a slice cut off for steak
- mela—rump
- petto—flank steak
- pezza—rump
- rosbif—roast beef
- scamone—rump
- spalla—chuck
- trippa—tripe
- vitellone magro—very lean baby beef

### *Agnello*—Lamb
- cosciotto—leg
- costata—rib
- costolette—loin chops
- peduccio—shank
- sella—loin roast
- spalla—shoulder

### *Maiale*—Pork
- braciole di maiale—pork chops
- cotolette di maiale—pork cutlets
- filetto di maiale—tenderloin
- porcellino di latte—suckling pig

*(continued on next page)*

**Dining Out**

**Italian**

## Cuts of Meat (continued)

*English—Italian*
**Poultry—*Pollame***

- capon—cappone
- chicken—pollo
  - breast—petto di pollo
  - leg—coscia di pollo
  - roast chicken—pollo arrosto
- duckling, duck—anitra
- goose—oca
- guinea hen—gallina faraona
- partridge—pernice
- pheasant—fagiano
- pigeon—piccione
- quail—quaglia
- turkey—tacchino
  - breast—petto di tacchino
  - leg—coscia di tacchino
  - roast turkey—tacchino arrosto
- wild duck—anitra selvatica

*Italian—English*
***Pollame*—Poultry**

- anitra—duckling, duck
- anitra selvatica—wild duck
- cappone—capon
- coscia di pollo—chicken leg
- coscia di tacchino—turkey leg
- fagiano—pheasant
- gallina faraona—guinea hen
- oca—goose
- pernice—partridge
- petto di pollo—chicken breast
- petto di tacchino—turkey breast
- piccione—pigeon
- pollo—chicken
- pollo arrosto—roast chicken
- quaglia—quail
- tacchino—turkey
- tacchino arrosto—roast turkey

**Veal—*Vitello***

- cutlets—cotolette
- leg—noce/girello/ controgirello/rosa/ soccoscio
- loin filet—filetto/lombata
- rib—petto/costola
- shank—muscolo
- shoulder—spalla

***Vitello*—Veal**

- controgirello—leg
- costola—rib
- cotolette—cutlets
- filetto—loin filet
- girello—leg
- lombata—loin filet
- muscolo—shank
- noce—leg
- petto—rib
- rosa—leg
- soccoscio—leg
- spalla—shoulder

*English—Italian*
**Other Meats You Might Enjoy**
- bacon—pancetta
- blood sausage— sanguinaccio
- brains—cervella
- chicken livers—fegatini di pollo
- goat/kid—capretto
- ham*—prosciutto/ prosciutto crudo/ prosciutto cotto
- kidneys—rognoni
- minced meat—carne tritata
- mutton—montone
- oxtail—codino di bue
- pig's feet—piedino di maiale
- rabbit—coniglio
- sausages—salsicce
- sweetbreads—animella
- tongue—lingua

*Italian—English*
- animella—sweetbreads
- capretto—goat/kid
- carne tritata—minced meat
- cervella—brains
- codino di bue—oxtail
- coniglio—rabbit
- fegatini di pollo— chicken livers
- lingua—tongue
- montone—mutton
- pancetta—bacon
- piedino di maiale—pig's feet
- prosciutto*—cured raw ham
- prosciutto cotto*— cooked ham
- prosciutto crudo*—cured raw ham
- rognoni—kidneys
- salsicce—sausages
- sanguinaccio—blood sausage

## Fish—Pesce and Shellfish—Crostacei

- **What kind of fish is this?**
  Che tipo di pesce è questo?

- **Please show me on this list.**
  Per favore, me lo indichi su quest'elenco.

*Cured but uncooked ham is very popular but also very expensive. You can select *prosciutto* or *prosciutto crudo*. Cooked ham is called *prosciutto cotto*.

■ **Is it fresh?**
È fresco?

■ **Has it been frozen? (You might want to know if what looks like fresh fish has actually been frozen and thawed.)**
È stato congelato?

■ **Do you have _____?**
Ha _____?

■ **I would like _____.**
Vorrei _____.

■ **Please give me _____.**
Per favore, mi dia _____.

# Fresh and Saltwater Fish

*English—Italian*
- anchovies—acciughe
  - fresh anchovies—alici
- angler fish (tail)—coda di rospo
- bass—branzino
- bream—pagello
- carp—carpa
- clams—vongole/arselle
- cod (dried, salted)—baccalà/stoccafisso
- crabs—granchi
- cuttlefish—seppie
- dogfish—palombo
- eel—anguilla/capitone
- flounder—passera
- grouper—spigola
- hake—nasello
- lobster (spiny)—aragosta
- mackerel—maccarello/sgombro

*Italian—English*
- acciughe—anchovies
- alici—fresh anchovies
- anguilla—eel
- aragosta—lobster (spiny)
- arselle—baby clams
- baccalà—dried salt cod
- branzino—bass
- calamari—squid
- capesante—scallops
- capitone—eel
- carpa—carp
- cefalo—gray mullet
- cernia—a game fish; considered a delicacy
- cicala di mare—lobster or prawnlike animal, minus the claws
- coda di rospo—tail of the angler fish
- cozze—mussels

## English—Italian

- mullet (gray)—cefalo
- mullet (red)—triglia
- mussels—cozze/mitili
- octopus—polipo
- perch (freshwater)—
  pesce persico
- perch (sea)—lupo di
  mare/occhiata
- pompanolike fish—
  dentice
- porgy—sarago
- prawns—mazzancolle/
  scampi
- sardines—sardine
  - fresh sardines—
    sarde
- scallops—capesante
- sea urchins—ricci
- shrimp—gamberi
  - large shrimp—
    gamberoni
- sole—sogliola
- squid—calamari/totani
- sturgeon—storione
- swordfish—pesce spada
- tench—tinca
- trout—trota
- tuna—tonno
- turbot—rombo

## Italian—English

- dentice—pompanolike
  fish
- gamberi—shrimp
- gamberoni—large shrimp
- granchi—crabs
- lupo di mare—sea perch
- maccarello—mackerel
- mazzancolle—prawns
- merluzzo—codfish
- mitili—mussels
- nasello—hake
- occhiata—fish in perch
  family
- ostriche—oysters
- pagello—bream
- palombo—dogfish
- passera—flounder
- pesce persico—perch
  (freshwater)
- pesce spada—swordfish
- polipo—octopus
- ricci—sea urchins
- rombo—turbot
- sarago—porgy
- sarde—fresh sardines
- sardine—sardines
- scampi—large shrimp/
  prawns
- scorfano—scorpion fish
  (rockfish)
- seppie—cuttlefish
- sgombro—mackerel
- sogliola—sole
- spigola—grouper
- stoccafisso—dried salt
  cod
- storione—sturgeon
- tartufi di mare—type
  of clam
- tinca—tench

*(continued on next page)*

**Dining Out**

**Italian**

# Fresh and Saltwater Fish
## (continued)

*English—Italian*

*Italian—English*
- tonno—tuna
- totani—squid
- triglie—red mullet
- trota—trout
- vongole—clams

# Vegetables—Legumi/Verdure

Frozen or canned vegetables are very rarely served in Italian restaurants, and you can count on fresh, in-season produce. The one exception will be the canned tomatoes occasionally used for stews and sauces.

- **Do you have _____?**
  Ha _____?

- **I would like _____.**
  Vorrei _____.

- **Please give me _____.**
  Per favore, mi dia _____.

# Vegetables

*English—Italian*
- artichokes—carciofi
- asparagus—asparagi
- beans—fagioli
  - broad beans—fave
  - green beans—fagiolini
- broccoli—broccoli
- brussels sprouts—broccoletti di Bruxelles
- cabbage—cavolo

*Italian—English*
- aglio—garlic
- aglio di serpe—chives
- asparagi—asparagus
- bietole—Swiss chard
- broccoletti di Bruxelles—brussels sprouts
- broccoli—broccoli
- capperi—capers
- carciofi—artichokes

## English—Italian

- red cabbage—cavolo rosso
- savoy cabbage—verza
- capers—capperi
- carrots—carote
- cauliflower—cavolfiore
- celery—sedano
- chick-peas—ceci
- chicory—cicoria
- chives—aglio di serpe
- corn on the cob—granturco
- cucumber—cetriolo
- eggplant—melanzana
- endive—indivia
- garlic—aglio
- leeks—porri
- lentils—lenticchie
- lettuce—lattuga
- mushrooms—funghi
- onions—cipolle
- parsley—prezzemolo
- parsnips—pastinache
- peas—piselli
- peppers—peperoni
  - red peppers—peperoncini
- potatoes—patate
- pumpkin—zucca
- radishes—ravanelli
- rice—riso
- spinach—spinaci
- Swiss chard—bietole
- tomatoes—pomodori
- truffles—tartufi
- turnips—rape
- zucchini—zucchini

## Italian—English

- carote—carrots
- cavolfiore—cauliflower
- cavolo—cabbage
- cavolo rosso—red cabbage
- ceci—chick-peas
- cicoria—chicory
- cipolle—onions
- fagioli—beans
- fagiolini—green beans
- fave—broad beans
- funghi—mushrooms
- granturco—corn on the cob
- indivia—endive
- lattuga—lettuce
- lenticchie—lentils
- melanzana—eggplant
- pastinache—parsnips
- patate—potatoes
- peperoncino—red pepper
- peperoni—peppers
- piselli—peas
- pomodori—tomatoes
- porri—leeks
- prezzemolo—parsley
- rape—turnips
- ravanelli—radishes
- riso—rice
- sedano—celery
- spinaci—spinach
- tartufi—truffles
- verza—savoy cabbage
- zucca—pumpkin
- zucchini—zucchini

# Pasta – Pasta

Pasta is eaten as a first course with almost all Italian meals. It is always cooked in salted water. If you're on a low-salt diet, ask:

■ **Please cook it in unsalted water.**
Per favore, lo faccia cuocere in acqua senza sale.

You may also need to know if the pasta contains any of the following ingredients. Ask:

■ **Please ask the chef to check the label on the container.**
Per favore, domandi allo chef di controllare l'etichetta sulla scatola.

■ **Does it contain _____?**
Contiene _____?
- egg (If you are allergic to egg, remember that many pasta noodles contain eggs.)—uovo
- salt—sale
- sugar—zucchero
- sweetening—dolcificante

### Types of Pasta
To describe all the pasta shapes and their uses would require more space than we have. Pasta can be made with:
- eggs—pasta all'uovo (Normally *fettuccine* or *tagliatelle* are made with eggs.)
- spinach—pasta verde (usually *fettuccine, tagliatelle* or *lasagne*)
- white flour (durum wheat)—farina bianca (grano duro)
- whole wheat flour—farina integrale
Full? Or ready for the next course?

# Nonalcoholic Beverages – Bevande Analcoliche

For fruit juices, see page 241.

For milk drinks, see page 247.
For coffee and tea, see pages 247–248.
Soft drinks are generally not available in restaurants, but you can get them at bars and snack bars. If you want a soft drink with a little less sugar than most, ask for a *gassosa,* something which is sold under several brand names. It comes in lemon and lime flavors. You might also try a homemade soft drink like orange juice mixed with soda water or lemonade.

■ **I would like _____.**
Vorrei _____.
  • lemonade (iced)—limonata con ghiaccio
  • orange juice with soda water—una spremuta d'arancia con acqua gassata
  • orange soda—aranciata
  • quinine-flavored soda (not tonic water)—chinotto

# Wine—Vino

■ **Please bring me a bottle of _____ wine.**
Per favore, mi porti una bottiglia di vino _____.

■ **I would like a liter (about a quart) of _____ wine.**
Vorrei un litro di vino _____.
  • abboccato—semisweet
  • bianco—white
  • de tavola—table (wine)
  • di casa—house (wine); usually excellent!
  • dolce—sweet
  • leggero—light
  • pastoso—full bodied
  • rosato—rosé
  • rosso—red
  • secco—dry
  • spumante—sparkling

# Part 3

## The Low-Sodium (Low-Salt) Diet

The following list of "not permitted" items may vary from the list of foods your physician has instructed you to avoid. To make the list easier for others to read, cross out the items that do not apply to you and add, PRINTING LEGIBLY, any other things you must avoid. Select them from the food lists on pages 239–257.

To make sure your food and drink are prepared properly, consult *Appendix 4: Italian Food Preparation.* Use it together with other appropriate pages when ordering meals.

Keep in mind that there are hidden sources of sodium in the food we eat. Baked goods, for instance, may be made with baking powder rather than yeast. Ask before you eat!

- **Is this made with yeast?**
  È preparato con lievito?

- **Is this made with baking powder/baking soda?**
  È preparato con lievito in polvere/bicarbonato di sodio?

Since *lievito* can refer to both yeast and the more general leavening, the *lievito* in a given product could be baking powder. So ask *both* of the preceding questions.

Another hidden source of salt is pasta, because it is always cooked in salted water. You must make a special request if you want your portion prepared in unsalted water. American-style baked potatoes? There are no such things in Italy. The closest relative is the *patate al forno,* which *is* oven-baked but also flavored with oil and spices; it is certain to contain salt. If you want plain baked potatoes, you had better call in ahead. (See pages 236–238.)

If you must keep to a diet of less than 800 milligrams of sodium a day, don't drink softened water. Ask!

- **Does this water/the water in the hotel pass through a filter that softens it/removes the hard minerals?**
  Quest 'acqua/l'acqua dell'albergo passa attraverso un filtro per renderla leggera/per rimuovere i minerali duri?

Also, check the labels on bottled water for its sodium content. Look for the word *sodio,* and remember that it may be part of a compound word. The bottled water table on page 27 should be consulted too. Note that *Fiuggi* brand water is low in sodium.

Beware also that antacids, like Alka Seltzer and other indigestion remedies, may contain sodium bicarbonate or another sodium compound. Before you go abroad, ask your physician to recommend a low-sodium antacid to take along. If you must buy an antacid overseas, here's the Italian for sodium bicarbonate or bicarbonate of soda: *bicarbonato di sodio.* Check the label for anything resembling the word *sodio.*

Finally, avoid anything containing capers, anchovies, and olives. They're all very, very salty!

So far, all you've read is *avoid, not permitted, beware,* and you're wondering what you can eat or drink in Italy and still stick to your diet. Unfortunately, your diet scenario will sound pretty negative too, but don't let that frighten you either. Take a look at the extensive food lists in *Part 2* of this section, pages 239–257. If you can't order from the menu the waiter gives you, ask for items on these food lists. Combine your selections with information from your diet scenario and *Appendix 4: Italian Food Preparation* to produce a satisfying meal, one custom-made to your specifications. Of course, there may be an extra charge for a request that takes an unusual amount of time to fulfill.

At last, the good news: frozen and canned vegetables are extremely rare in Italian restaurants. The vegetables on the menu are likely to be those in season. But to be sure, ask before you order. The exceptions to this rule are tomatoes. In many parts of Italy, tomatoes are cooked, crushed, and canned routinely, because they provide the necessary ingredient in so many dishes. Tomatoes go out of season, but, in Italy, red sauces do not. Fortunately, tomatoes are often canned without salt. Often, but not always. Ask!

---

# Foods Not Permitted — Sostanze/Cibi Vietati

- anchovies—acciughe
- anything prepared with baking powder or with baking soda—qualsiasi cosa preparata con bicarbonato di sodio
- baking soda—bicarbonato di sodio
- bouillon—consommé
- broth—brodo
- canned fish—pesce in scatola
- canned meat—carne in scatola
- canned tomatoes—pomodori in scatola
- canned vegetables—legumi/verdure in scatola
- capers—capperi
- catsup—ketchup americano
- cheese—formaggio
- chive—aglio di serpe
- condensed milk—latte condensato
- cured meats—salumi
- garlic salt—sale d'aglio
- gravy—sugo/salsa di carne
- instant or frozen potatoes—patate surgelate
- margarine—margarina
- mayonnaise—maionese
- meat sauce—salsa in bottiglia per carni
- milk—latte
- monosodium glutamate (MSG)—glutamato di monosodio
- mustard—mostarda
- olives—olive
- pickled vegetables—sottaceti
- salt—sale
- salted butter—burro salato
- salted salad dressing—condimenti per insalata preparati con sale
- sauces with bacon drippings—sughi/condimenti preparati con guanciale o pancetta
- sausage—salsiccia
- sodium preservatives—conservanti contenenti sodio
- soy sauce—salsa di soia
- tomato puree—pomodori passati
- tomato sauce—sugo di pomodoro

---

# The Low-Sodium (Low-Salt) Scenario

If you can't pronounce the Italian, point to appropriate phrases. For some sample replies to your questions, turn to *Appendix 4: Italian Food Preparation* and show it to your respondent.

■ **I have a reservation. My name is _____.**
Ho una prenotazione. Mi chiamo _____.

■ **Please tell the manager I am here.**
Per favore, dica al direttore che sono qui.

■ **The manager knows about the special service I need because of a medical problem.**
Il direttore è al corrente del riguardo speciale di cui ho bisogno per un problema medico.

■ **Does anyone here speak English?**
C'è nessuno qui che parli inglese?

■ **I/she/he must follow a special diet.**
Devo/deve seguire una dieta speciale.

■ **All food and drink must be completely salt-free.**
Tutto il cibo e le bevande devono essere completamente senza sale.

■ **Everything must be prepared without the foods/substances on this list.**
Tutto deve essere preparato senza i cibi/le sostanze su questo elenco.

■ **A mistake can cause serious illness.**
Un errore può provocare una grave malattia.

■ **Does this dish contain any salt?**
C'è sale in questo piatto?

■ **Does this dish contain anything on this list?**
Nel piatto c'è qualcosa su questo elenco?

- **Can you prepare this dish without salt/sauce?**
Può preparare questo piatto senza sale/salsa?

- **Can you prepare this dish without any of the items on this list?**
Può preparare questo piatto senza le sostanze su questo elenco?

- **Show me on the menu which dishes you can prepare without salt?**
Mi indichi sulla lista quali piatti può preparare senza sale.

- **Show me on the menu which dishes you can prepare without any of the items on this list?**
Mi indichi sulla lista quali piatti può preparare senza le sostanze su questo elenco.

- **Which dishes on the menu are salt-free?**
Quali piatti sulla lista sono senza sale?

- **Are there any dishes on the menu that do not contain ingredients forbidden to me?**
Ci sono piatti sulla lista che non contengono gli ingredienti che mi sono vietati?

- **Are the tomatoes in this dish fresh, frozen, or canned? (Please point to the right word.)**
I pomodori in questo piatto sono freschi, surgelati, o in scatola? (Per favore, mi indichi la parola giusta.)

- **Can you prepare a serving of pasta for me, cooked in unsalted water?**
Mi può preparare una porzione di pastasciutta cotta in acqua senza sale?

- **Are the potatoes/vegetables cooked in salted water?**
Le patate/le verdure sono cotte in acqua salata?

- **Can you prepare potatoes/vegetables for me, cooked in unsalted water?**

Mi può preparare una porzione di patate/verdure cotte in acqua senza sale?

- **If you are not sure, please tell me/ask the chef/the maitre d'.**

Se non è sicuro, per favore me lo dica/lo chieda allo chef/al maitre d'hotel.

- **I would like to speak to the chef/the maitre d'.**

Vorrei parlare allo chef/al maitre d'hotel.

- **Can you prepare something simple for me in your kitchen that is salt-free? For example, baked or broiled fish without seasoning/sauces; steak; baked, boiled, or mashed potatoes; fresh, cooked, unsalted vegetables? Potatoes and vegetables must be cooked in unsalted water.**

Potrebbe prepararmi qualche piatto semplice in cucina che sia senza sale? Per esempio, pesce al forno o in graticola senza condimenti/salse; bistecca; patate al forno, bollite o puré; verdure/legumi freschi, cotti, senza sale? Le patate e le verdure/i legumi devono essere cotti in acqua senza sale.

- **Do you have a microwave oven/a pressure cooker?**

Ha un forno a microonde/una pentola a pressione?

(If the answer is *yes,* then ask:)

- **Can you prepare a single portion of _____, plain/without seasoning/gravy/sauce/salt?**

Mi può preparare una porzione di _____, semplice/senza condimenti/sugo/salsa/sale?

- **A mistake has been made. This is not what I ordered.**

È stato fatto un errore. Non è questo che ho ordinato.

# The Diabetic Diet

Your physician has outlined a diet for you and probably shown you how to select balanced meals using a system of food exchanges. The phrases in this section will help you identify dishes on a menu that contain added sweetening. If you must also observe a low-fat, low-cholesterol diet, refer to the low-fat, low-cholesterol scenario.

**Caution:** If you must take an antacid, be sure to read the information on page 15 about the sugar content of many popular antacids.

To make sure your food is properly prepared, consult *Appendix 4: Italian Food Preparation.* Use it together with other appropriate pages when ordering meals.

Artificial sweeteners are not available in most Italian restaurants. If you want to carry an artificial sweetener for use in coffee or tea, try a pharmacy. Food products for diabetics are also sold in most pharmacies.

Check the "not permitted" list. To make it easier for others to read, cross out the items that do not apply to you and add things you cannot have. PRINT LEGIBLY! Select them from the food lists on pages 239–257.

---

## Foods Not Permitted – Sostanze/Cibi Vietati

- barley syrup—sciroppo di orzo
- butter—burro
- condensed milk—latte condensato
- corn syrup—sciroppo di mais
- dextrose—destrosio
- fats—grassi
- fructose—fruttosio/levulosio
- honey—miele
- jam and marmalade—marmellata
- jelly—gelatina di frutta
- lard—lardo
- maltose—maltosio
- margarine—margarina
- molasses—melassa
- oils—oli
- rice syrup—sciroppo di riso
- shortening—grassi per pasticceria
- sugar—zucchero
- syrup—sciroppo

---

# The Diabetic Scenario

If you can't pronounce the Italian, point to the appropriate phrases. For some sample replies to your questions, turn to *Appendix 4: Italian Food Preparation* and show it to your respondent.

- **I have a reservation. My name is _____.**
  Ho una prenotazione. Mi chiamo _____.

- **Please tell the manager that I am here.**
  Per favore, dica al direttore che sono qui.

- **The manager knows about the special service I need because of a medical problem.**
  Il direttore è al corrente del riguardo speciale di cui ho bisogno per un problema medico.

- **Does anyone here speak English?**
  C'è nessuno qui che parli inglese?

- **I/she/he must follow a special diet because of diabetes.**
  Devo/deve seguire una dieta speciale per la diabete.

- **All food and drink must be free of added sugar or sweetening.**
  Tutto il cibo e le bevande devono essere senza aggiunta di zucchero o dolcificanti.

- **Everything must be prepared without the ingredients on this list.**
  Tutto deve essere preparato senza gli ingredienti su questo elenco.

- **A mistake can cause serious illness.**
  Un errore può provocare una grave malattia.

Diabetic Diet

Italian

- **Does this dish/beverage/juice contain any of the substances on this list?**
Questo piatto/bevanda/succo contiene uno dei dolcificanti sull'elenco?

- **Can you prepare this dish/beverage/juice without sweetening?**
Può preparare questo piatto/bevanda/succo senza dolcificanti?

- **Are the fruits/vegetables in this dish fresh/canned/frozen?**
La frutta/verdure/legumi in questo piatto sono freschi/in scatola/surgelati?

- **If it is canned or frozen in syrup, please drain all the liquid.**
Se sono in scatola o surgelati in uno sciroppo, per favore faccia scolare tutto il liquido.

- **Do you have any artificial sweetener?**
Ha un dolcificante artificiale?

- **If you are not sure, please tell me/ask the chef/the maitre d'.**
Se non è sicuro, per favore me lo dica/lo chieda allo chef/al maitre d'hotel.

- **I would like to speak to the chef/the maitre d'.**
Vorrei parlare allo chef/al maitre d'hotel.

- **Do you have a microwave oven/a pressure cooker?**
Ha un forno a microonde/una pentola a pressione?

(If the answer is *yes*, then ask:)

- **Can you prepare a single portion of _____, without seasoning/gravy/sauce/sugar/sweetening?**
Mi può preparare una porzione di _____, senza condimenti/sugo/salsa/zucchero/dolcificante.

■ **A mistake has been made. This is not what I ordered.**
È stato fatto un errore. Non è questo che ho ordinato.

# The Low-Fat and Low-Cholesterol Diet

The following list of "not-permitted" items may vary from the foods your physician has instructed you to avoid. To make the list easier for others to read, cross out the items that do not apply to you, and write in, PRINTING LEGIBLY, the things you must avoid. Select them from the food lists on pages 239–257.

To make sure your food and drinks are prepared properly, consult *Appendix 4: Italian Food Preparation.* Use it together with other appropriate pages when ordering meals.

Happily for you, meat in Italy is lean. Beef is slaughtered young and generally sold with most of the fat trimmed away. It is more expensive that way, but there is also less waste. American-style, marbled meat is non-existent: Italians like their meat very lean. Nor is meat aged as it is in the United States. Baby veal and veal are the most popular varieties. In fact, even American veal is older than Italian veal.

Baked potatoes to go with that lean meat? In Italy there is no such thing as an American-style baked potato. In the nearest thing to an equivalent dish, *patate al forno,* potatoes are usually oven-baked with oil and spices. So, if you want the dish without oil, you must ask for changes in the recipe.

---

## Foods Not Permitted — Sostanze/Cibi Vietati

- all animal fats—qualsiasi grasso animale
- all fats—qualsiasi grasso
- all oils—qualsiasi olio
- avocado—avocado
- bacon fat—grasso di pancetta/guanciale
- butter—burro
- canned meat/fish—carne/ pesce in scatola

*(continued on next page)*

## Foods Not Permitted –
## Sostanze/Cibi Vietati (continued)

- cheese sauces—salse a base di formaggio
- chocolate—cioccolato
- cocoa—cacao
- cocoa butter—burro di cacao
- coconut—noce di cocco
- coconut oil—olio di noce di cocco
- cream—panna
- eggs—uova
- egg yolk—tuorlo d'uovo
- fried foods—cibi fritti
- gravy—sugo
- ground meat—carne tritata
- heart—cuore
- hydrogenated oil—oli idrogenizzati
- kidney—rognone
- lard—lardo
- liver—fegato
- margarine—margarina
- mayonnaise—maionese

- nuts—noci
- olive oil—olio d'oliva
- palm kernel oil—olio di semi di palma
- palm oil—olio di palma
- part skim milk—latte parzialmente scremato
- peanut oil—olio di arachidi
- salad dressing oil— condimenti per insalata a base di olio
- sausage—salsiccia
- sauce—salsa
- shortening—grassi per pasticceria
- shrimp—gamberi
- sweetbreads—animella
- whole milk—latte intero
- whole or part skim milk/ cheese/yogurt—formaggio o yogurt fatto di latte intero o parzialmente scremato

## The Low-Fat and Low-Cholesterol Scenario

If you can't pronounce the Italian, point to the appropriate phrases. For some sample replies to your questions, turn to *Appendix 4: Italian Food Preparation* and show it to your respondent.

- **I have a reservation. My name is _____.**
Ho una prenotazione. Mi chiamo _____.

- **Please tell the manager that I am here.**
Per favore, dica al direttore che sono qui.

- **The manager knows about the special service I need because of a medical problem.**

Il direttore è al corrente del riguardo speciale di cui ho bisogno per un problema medico.

- **Does anyone here speak English?**

C'è nessuno qui che parli inglese?

- **I/she/he must follow a special diet because of a serious medical problem.**

Devo/deve seguire una dieta speciale per un grave problema medico.

- **All food and drink must be fat-free.**

Tutto il cibo e le bevande devono essere senza grassi.

- **Everything must be prepared without the ingredients on this list.**

Tutto deve essere preparato senza gli ingredienti su questo elenco.

- **Nothing can be fried.**

Niente può essere fritto.

- **All visible fat must be trimmed before cooking.**

Tutto il grasso visibile deve essere rimosso prima della cottura.

- **A mistake can cause serious illness.**

Un errore può provocare una grave malattia.

- **Does this dish contain any _____?**

Questo piatto contiene _____?

- **Can you prepare this dish without _____?**

Può preparare questo piatto senza _____?

- **Can you prepare this dish with _____ instead of _____?**
Può preparare questo piatto con _____ invece di _____?

- **Does this dish contain anything on this list?**
Questo piatto contiene qualcosa su questo elenco?

- **Can you prepare this dish without any of the items on this list?**
Può preparare questo piatto senza gli ingredienti su questo elenco?

- **Are there any dishes on your menu that do not contain ingredients forbidden to me?**
Ci sono piatti sulla lista che non contengono le sostanze che mi sono vietate?

- **Can you fry/prepare this dish with any of these oils: safflower/sunflower/corn/soy/cottonseed/peanut?**
Può friggere/preparare questo piatto senza questi oli: olio di cartamo/olio di semi di girasole/olio di mais/olio di semi di soia/olio di semi di cotone/olio di arachidi?

- **Please prepare this dish without any sauce/gravy.**
Per favore, prepari questo piatto senza sugo/salsa.

- **If you are not sure, please tell me/ask the chef/the maitre d'.**
Se non è sicuro, per favore me lo dica/domandi allo chef/al direttore.

- **I would like to speak to the chef/the maitre d'.**
Vorrei parlare allo chef/al maitre d'hotel.

- **Do you have a microwave oven/a pressure cooker?**
Ha un forno a microonde/una pentola a pressione?

(If the answer is *yes*, then ask:)

- **Can you prepare a single portion of _____, plain/without seasoning/gravy/sauce/butter/oil/fats?**
  Mi può preparare una porzione di _____, semplice/ senza condimenti/sugo/salse/burro/olio/grassi?

- **A mistake has been made. This is not what I ordered.**
  È stato fatto un errore. Non è questo che ho ordinato.

# The Ulcer, Bland, Soft, and Low-Residue Diet

The items on the following list may vary from the foods your physician has instructed you to avoid. To make the list easier for others to read, cross out the items that do not apply to you and write in, PRINTING LEGIBLY, the things you cannot have. Select them from the food lists on pages 239–257.

To make sure your food and beverage are prepared properly, consult *Appendix 4: Italian Food Preparation.* Use it together with other appropriate pages when ordering meals.

## Foods Not Permitted – Sostanze/Cibi Vietati

- bran—crusca
- brown/wild rice—riso integrale/selvatico
- catsup—ketchup americano
- clams—vongole
- coarse bread—pane cafone (preparato senza farina raffinata)
- coarse cereals—cereali grossi
- coconut—noce di cocco
- corn—granturco
- dried fruits—frutta essiccata
- dried legumes—verdure/ ortaggi essiccati
- fat—grasso
- foods prepared with wine or liqueurs—piatti preparati con vino o liquori
- fried foods—cibi fritti
- garlic—aglio
- gravy—sugo

*(continued on next page)*

## Foods Not Permitted —
## Sostanze/Cibi Vietati (continued)

- herbs—odori/erbe
- lard—lardo
- meat broth—brodo di carne
- mustard—mostarda
- nuts/seeds—noci/semi
- olives—olive
- onions—cipolle
- oysters—ostriche
- paprika—paprica
- peas—piselli
- pepper—pepe
- pickled meat/fish—salumi/ pesce conservato sotto aceto

- pickled vegetables— sottaceti
- pork—carne suina
- raisins—uva passa
- red pepper—peperoncino forte
- salt—sale
- sauce—sugo
- seasoning—condimenti
- sharp (strong) cheese— formaggio forte
- spices—spezie
- vinegar—aceto

# The Ulcer, Bland, Soft, and Low-Residue Scenario

If you cannot pronounce the Italian, point to appro-priate phrases. For some sample replies to your questions, turn to *Appendix 4: Italian Food Preparation* and show it to your respondent.

- **I have a reservation. My name is _____.**

Ho una prenotazione. Mi chiamo _____.

- **Please tell the manager I am here.**

Per favore dica al direttore che sono qui.

- **The manager knows about the special service I need because of a medical problem.**

Il direttore è al corrente del riguardo speciale di cui ho bisogno per un problema medico.

- **Does anyone here speak English?**

C'è nessuno qui che parli inglese?

- **I/she/he must follow a special diet for a stomach problem.**
Devo/deve seguire una dieta speciale per un problema medico allo stomaco.

- **Everything must be prepared without spices/seasoning.**
Tutti i piatti devono essere preparati senza spezie/condimenti.

- **Please, no fried foods. Food must be baked/broiled/stewed/poached.**
Per favore, niente cibi fritti. I piatti devono essere preparati al forno/alla griglia/in umido/bolliti.

- **A mistake can cause serious illness.**
Un errore può provocare una grave malattia.

- **Please bake/broil/stew/poach this dish.**
Per favore, prepari al forno/alla griglia/in umido/come bollito/questo piatto.

- **Can you bake/broil/stew/poach/this dish?**
Può preparare al forno/alla griglia/in umido/come bollito/questo piatto?

- **Everything must be prepared without the ingredients on this list. Please read it. Thank you.**
Tutto deve essere preparato senza gli ingredienti su questo elenco. Lo legga per favore. Grazie.

- **Does this dish contain any _____?**
Questo piatto contiene _____?

- **Can you prepare this dish without _____?**
Può preparare questo piatto senza _____?

■ **Can you prepare this dish with _____ instead of _____?**
Può preparare questo piatto con _____ invece di _____?

■ **If you are not sure, please tell me/ask the chef/the maitre d'.**
Se non è sicuro, per favore me lo dica/domandi allo chef/al maitre d'hotel.

■ **Can you prepare something bland and simple like a platter of plain baked fish, baked potato without oil or fats, or plain boiled potatoes/tender carrots/spinach/green beans/ mushrooms?**
Mi può preparare qualcosa di semplice, senza condimenti, come una porzione di pesce al forno, patate al forno (senza olio o grassi) o bollite/carote bollite/ spinaci/fagiolini/funghi?

■ **Do you have a microwave oven/a pressure cooker?**
Ha un forno a microonde/una pentola a pressione?

(If the answer is *yes,* then ask:)

■ **Can you prepare a single portion of _____, plain, without seasoning/gravy/sauce?**
Mi può preparare una porzione di _____, semplice/ senza condimenti/sugo/salse?

■ **A mistake has been made. This is not what I ordered.**
È stato fatto un errore. Non è questo che ho ordinato.

■ **I would like to speak to the chef/the maitre d'.**
Vorrei parlare allo chef/al maitre d'hotel.

# Design Your Own Scenario for a Custom-made Diet

If, for health, personal, or religious reasons you require a special diet and it does not appear in our repertoire, you can produce your own script. We've made it easy for you by supplying the phrases on the following pages. To fill in the blanks of the various phrases, do the following:

**1.** On a separate sheet of paper, prepare a list of foods that you cannot eat.

**2.** To translate your list into Italian, use the "not permitted" lists under the other diets and the food lists on pages 239–257; you might also find the supplementary items at the end of this chapter useful.

**3.** Copy your list into this book, PRINTING LEGIBLY, in the blank spaces provided under the heading, "not permitted." PRINT it in English *and* Italian.

**4.** PRINT the Italian words, where applicable, in the blanks in the script.

**5.** Of course, don't forget to use *Appendix 4: Italian Food Preparation* to explain how you want your food prepared.

| Foods Not Permitted | Sostanze/ Cibi Vietati |
|---|---|
| | |
| | |
| | |
| | |
| | |
| | |
| | |
| | |
| | |
| | |
| | |
| | |
| | |
| | |
| | |
| | |
| | |

# The Custom-made Scenario

If you can't pronounce the Italian, point to the appropriate phrases. For some sample replies to your questions, turn to *Appendix 4: Italian Food Preparation* and show it to your respondent.

- **I have a reservation. My name is _____.**
  Ho una prenotazione. Mi chiamo _____.

- **Please tell the manager I am here.**
  Per favore, dica al direttore che sono qui.

- **The manager knows about the special service I need because of a medical problem.**
  Il direttore è al corrente del riguardo speciale di cui ho bisogno per un problema medico.

- **The manager knows about the special diet I need.**
  Il direttore è al corrente della dieta speciale di cui ho bisogno.

- **Does anyone here speak English?**
  C'è nessuno qui che parli inglese?

- **I/she/he must follow a special diet.**
  Devo/deve seguire una dieta speciale.

- **All food and drink must be prepared without _____.**
  Tutto il cibo e le bevande devono essere preparate senza _____.

- **Everything must be prepared without the substances/ingredients on this list.**
  Tutto deve essere preparato senza le sostanze/ingredienti su questo elenco.

- **A mistake can cause serious illness.**

  Un errore può provocare una grave malattia.

- **Does this dish contain any _____?**

  Qúesto piatto contiene _____?

- **Does this dish contain anything on this list?**

  Questo piatto contiene qualcosa su quest'elenco?

- **Can you prepare this dish without _____?**

  Può preparare questo piatto senza _____?

- **Show me on the menu which dishes you can prepare without _____.**

  Mi indichi sulla lista quali piatti può preparare senza _____.

- **Show me on the menu which dishes you can prepare without any of the items on this list.**

  Mi indichi sulla lista quali piatti può preparare senza le sostanze/gli ingredienti su quest'elenco.

- **Are there any dishes on the menu that do not contain ingredients forbidden to me?**

  Ci sono piatti sulla lista che non contengono ingredienti che mi sono vietati?

- **If you are not sure, please tell me/ask the chef/the maitre d'.**

  Se non è certo, per favore me lo dica/lo chieda allo chef/al maitre d'hotel.

- **I would like to speak to the chef/the maitre d'.**

  Vorrei parlare allo chef/al maitre d'hotel.

- **Can you prepare something simple for me in your kitchen that is appropriate for my diet? For example: _____.**

  Mi può preparare in cucina qualcosa di semplice che sia accettabile per la mia dieta? Per esempio: _____.

Custom-made Diet

Italian

- **Do you have a microwave oven/a pressure cooker?**
Ha un forno a microonde/una pentola a pressione?

(If the answer is *yes,* then ask:)

- **Can you prepare a single portion of _____ without _____?**
Può prepararmi una porzione di _____ senza _____?

- **A mistake has been made. This is not what I ordered.**
È stato fatto un errore. Non è questo che ho ordinato.

To compose a list of forbidden items, consult the food lists on pages 239–257, the collection of no-nos for the other scenarios, and this sampling of foods that may cause reactions in some allergenic and otherwise sensitive individuals.

## Possible Forbidden Items – Sostanze/Cibi Vietati

- barley—orzo
- barley cereal—cereali d'orzo
- barley flour—farina d'orzo
- beef/veal—manzo/vitello
- beets—barbabietole
- bran—crusca
- buckwheat—grano saraceno
- buckwheat cereal—cereali di grano saraceno
- buckwheat flour—farina di grano saraceno
- buckwheat stuffing—ripieno a base di grano saraceno
- chocolate—cioccolato
- cinnamon—cannella
- citrus fruits—agrumi
- coconut—noce di cocco
- coffee—caffè
- cola—bevande tipo Coca-Cola, Pepsi-Cola, etc.
- corn—granturco
- corn products—prodotti di granturco
- dates—datteri
- eggs—uova
- figs—fichi
- fish—pesce
- flaxseed—semi di lino
- fresh beans—fagioli freschi
- legumes—legumi
- lettuce—lattuga
- malt—malto
- malt flavoring—cibi/bevande aromatizzati con malto
- milk—latte
- nuts—noci

- oat flour—farina d'avena
- oatmeal bread—pane di farina d'avena
- oatmeal cereal—cereali di farina d'avena
- oatmeal stuffing—ripieno a base di avena
- oats—avena
- peanuts—arachidi (noccioline americane)
- pork—suino
- potato—patate
- rice—riso
- rye—segale
- rye bread—pane di segale
- rye bread crumbs—pangrattato di segale
- rye cereal—cereali di segale
- rye flour—farina di segale
- shellfish—frutti di mare/ crostacei
- soybeans—semi di soia
- string beans—fagiolini
- sugar (cane)—canna da zucchero
- tomato—pomodoro
- wheat—frumento
- wheat bread—pane di frumento
- wheat cereal—cereali di frumento
- wheat crumbs—pangrattato di frumento
- wheat flour—farina di frumento
- wheat germ—germoglio di frumento
- wheat stuffing—ripieno a base di frumento
- yeast—lievito

Custom-made Diet

Italian

# Medical Aid

Read these pages now. They will make things easier for you later.

In an acute emergency ask an Italian-speaking person to telephone for help for you. You will find the phrase for such a request under *Emergencies,* on page 284. Memorize it now.

## U.S. Embassy and Consular Assistance in Italy

If you are visiting Rome, you can obtain a list of qualified English-speaking physicians from the American Embassy. It's a good thing to keep handy. Why wait for an emergency? Get your umbrella before it rains! When in Rome, pick up the list at the:

**Embassy of the United States**, Via Vittorio Veneto 119/A. Telephone: area code (06)-4674.

Consular services are available in other Italian cities, too:

**Florence** — Lungarno Amerigo Vespucci 38. Telephone: area code (055) 29 82 76.

**Genoa** — Banca d'America e d'Italia Building, Centralino Piazza Portello 6. Telephone: area code (010) 28 27/41 or 42/43/44/45.

**Milan** — Piazza della Repubblica 32. Telephone: area code (02) 65 28/41 or 42/43/44/45.

**Naples** — Piazza della Repubblica. Telephone: area code (081) 66 09 66.

**Trieste** — Via Roma 9 (4th floor). Telephone: area code (040) 687 28 or 29.

# Emergencies

■ **Help!**
  Aiuto!

- **Police!**
  Polizia!

- **Fire!**
  Incendio!

- **I am ill.**
  Mi sento male.

- **She/he is ill.**
  Si sente male.

- **Call a doctor right away.**
  Chiami subito un dottore.

- **Call an ambulance right away.**
  Chiami subito uń ambulanza.

- **Take me/us to a doctor right away.**
  Mi/ci porti subito da un dottore.

- **Take me/us to a hospital right away.**
  Mi/ci porti subito a un ospedale.

- **Is there a doctor in the building?**
  C'è un dottore in questo edificio?

- **I cannot speak Italian. Please call this number for me.**
  Non so parlare italiano. Per favore, chiami per me questo numero.

# Emergency Telephone Numbers

When you check in at your lodgings, ask the clerk or manager for emergency numbers. Of course you'll feel foolish making such a request before you've even seen your room or unpacked your bags. But no matter. Try out these phrases, and when you've got the numbers, fill in the blanks of the *Emergency Telephone Numbers* box below. Or better yet, ask the clerk to fill it in for you. If you show him or her the book with this official-looking box, your request won't appear so strange after all.

■ **I would like emergency numbers in this box. Would you mind filling it in for me? Thank you.**

Vorrei numeri da chiamare in caso di emergenza in questo riquadro. Le dispiacerebbe scrivermeli? Grazie.

---

**Emergency Telephone Numbers—**
**Numeri da Chiamare in Caso di Emergenza**

Ambulance—Ambulanza: _____

Fire—Vigili del Fuoco: _____

Police—Polizia: _____

---

# Asking for Help

■ **Where is the nearest doctor?**
Dov' è il dottore piú vicino?

- **Where is the nearest hospital/clinic?**
  Dov' e il piú vicino ospedale/clinica?

- **Where is the nearest first-aid station?**
  Dov'è il piú vicino pronto soccorso?

- **Where is the nearest pharmacy?**
  Dov'è la farmacia piú vicina?

- **Where is the nearest English-speaking doctor?**
  Dov'è il piú vicino dottore che parla inglese?

- **Is there an English-speaking doctor here?**
  C'è un dottore che parla inglese qui?

- **Is there a hospital here with English-speaking doctors?**
  C'è un ospedale qui con dottori che parlano inglese?

- **At what time can the doctor come?**
  A che ora può venire il dottore?

- **What are the office hours?**
  Qual è l'orario d'ufficio?

- **Please PRINT the information. Thank you.**
  Per favore, scriva in STAMPATELLO le informazioni. Grazie.

- **What is the doctor's name, address, and telephone number?**
  Qual è il nome del dottore, il suo indirizzo e numero telefonico?

- **Please show me where it is on this map.**
  Per favore, mi indichi dov'è su questa cartina.

**■ Please show me on this map where we are now.**
Per favore, mi indichi su questa cartina dove siamo ora.

**■ Please draw a map/sketch for me.**
Per favore, mi disegni una cartina/mi faccia un disegnino.

**■ I cannot speak Italian. Please phone for me.**
Non so parlare italiano. Per favore, telefoni per me.

**■ Does anyone here speak English?**
C'è nessuno qui che parli inglese?

**■ I need an interpreter.**
Ho bisogno di un interprete.

# Numbers

| | |
|---|---|
| 0 — zero | 31 — trentuno |
| 1 — uno, una | 38 — trentotto |
| 2 — due | 40 — quaranta |
| 3 — tre | 50 — cinquanta |
| 4 — quattro | 60 — sessanta |
| 5 — cinque | 70 — settanta |
| 6 — sei | 80 — ottanta |
| 7 — sette | 90 — novanta |
| 8 — otto | 100 — cento |
| 9 — nove | 101 — centouno |
| 10 — dieci | 200 — duecento |
| 11 — undici | 300 — trecento |
| 12 — dodici | 400 — quattrocento |
| 13 — tredici | 500 — cinquecento |
| 14 — quattordici | 1000 — mille |
| 15 — quindici | 2000 — duemila |
| 16 — sedici | 3000 — tremila |
| 17 — diciasette | 10,000 — diecimila |
| 18 — diciotto | 20,000 — ventimila |
| 19 — diciannove | 100,000 — centomila |
| 20 — venti | 500,000 — cinquecentomila |
| 21 — ventuno | 1,000,000 — un milione |
| 22 — ventidue | half — mezzo |
| 28 — ventotto | quarter — un quarto di |
| 30 — trenta | |

# Appendix 1:
# Spanish Food Preparation

## How to Make Sure Your Food Is Properly Prepared

■ **Please, I would like this dish _____.**

Este platillo lo quiero _____ por favor.
- baked—asado
- boiled—hervido
- broiled/grilled—a la parrilla
- cold—frío
- fried—frito
- hot—caliente
- medium—a punto (S)*, termino medio (M)
- poached—escalfado
- rare—poco asado
- roasted—al horno
- sautéed—reogado (S), salteado (M)
- steamed— al vapor
- well done—bien asado (S), bien hecho (M)
- with all visible fat trimmed before cooking—con toda la grasa visible recortada antes de cocinar

■ **Please, I would like it with/without _____.**

Por favor, quiero este platillo con/sin _____.

■ **Please serve the _____ in a separate dish.**

Por favor, sírvame el/la _____ en otro plato.
- black pepper—pimienta
- butter (unsalted)—mantequilla (sin sal)
- chilies—guindillas (S), chiles (M)
- cream—crema (M), nata (S)
- dressing—aderezo
- fresh skim milk—leche fresca descremada
- margarine—margarina
- saccharin—sacarina
- salt—sal

*(M) = Mexico; (S) = Spain

- sauce/gravy—salsa
- seasoning—condimentos
- spices—especias
- stuffing—relleno
- sugar—azúcar
- sweetening—endulzante
- whole milk—leche entera

# Possible Replies

■ **Mr./Ms./Waiter/Manager/Maitre D': Please, point to your reply. Thank you.**

Señor/Señora/Mozo (S), Mesero (M)/Sr. Gerente/ Maitre: Haga el favor de mostrarme su respuesta, gracias.

■ **I understand but cannot help you.**

Comprendo, pero no puedo ayudarle.

■ **I can prepare it as you wish.**

Se lo puedo preparar como usted guste.

■ **Wait, I'll ask the chef/the maitre d'.**

Espere, le preguntaré al chef/al maitre.

■ **If you can wait a while, we can prepare it as you wish.**

Si puede usted esperar un momento, se lo podemos preparar como usted guste.

■ **With sufficient notice we can prepare a special dish for you. We need:**

Con aviso de ante mano, le podremos preparar un platillo especial. Necesitaremos saberlo con:
- 3 or 4 hours notice—3 o 4 horas de anticipo
- 24 hours notice—24 horas de anticipo
- 2 days notice—2 días de anticipo

■ **Wait, I'll get someone who speaks English.**

Espere, voy por alguien que hable inglés.

# Appendix 2:
# German Food Preparation

## How to Make Sure Your Food Is Properly Prepared

- **I would like it _____.**
  Ich hätte es bitte gern _____.
    - baked—gebacken
    - boiled—gekocht
    - broiled—auf dem Rost gebraten
    - cold—kalt
    - fried—pfannengebraten
    - grilled—gegrillt
    - hot—heiss
    - medium—halbdurch
    - rare—roh, innen rot
    - roasted—im Ofen gebraten
    - sautéed—sautiert
    - steamed—gedämpft
    - well done—ganz durch
    - with all fat trimmed before cooking—mit allem Fett vor dem Kochen abgeschnitten; ohne jegliches Fett

- **I would like it with/without _____.**
  Ich hätte es bitte gern mit/ohne _____.
    - black pepper—Pfeffer
    - butter (without salt)—Butter (ohne Salz)
    - chilies—Chili
    - cream—Sahne
    - dressing—Salatsauce
    - fresh milk—frischer Milch
    - gravy—Sosse
    - margarine—Margarine
    - saccharin—künstlichem Süssstoff
    - salt—Salz
    - sauce—Sauce

- seasoning—Gewürze
- skim milk—Magermilch
- stuffing—Füllung
- sugar—Zucker
- sweetening—süssen Zutaten, Süssmacher

# Possible Replies

- **Ms./Mr./Waiter/Maitre D': Please point to your reply. Thank you.**
Fräulein/Herr/Ober/Oberkellner: Bitte zeigen Sie auf Ihre Antwort. Vielen Dank.

- **I understand but cannot help you.**
Ich verstehe, aber ich kann leider nichts für Sie tun.

- **I can prepare it as you wish.**
Es kann so, wie Sie es möchten, zubereitet werden.

- **Wait, I'll ask the chef/the maitre d'.**
Einen Moment, ich frage den Koch/den Oberkellner.

- **If you can wait a while, we can prepare it as you wish.**
Wenn Sie etwas warten, können wir es so zubereiten, wie Sie es möchten.

- **With sufficient notice we can prepare a special dish for you. We need:**
Wenn Sie uns lange genug im voraus benachrichtigen, können wir ein besonderes Essen für Sie zubereiten. Wir brauchen Ihre Bestellung:
  - 3 or 4 hours notice—3 oder 4 Stunden im voraus
  - 24 hours notice—24 Stunden im voraus
  - 2 days notice— 2 Tage im voraus

- **Wait, I'll get someone who speaks English.**
Einen Moment, ich hole jemanden, der Englisch spricht.

German

German Food Preparation

289

# Appendix 3:
# French Food Preparation

## How to Make Sure Your Food Is Properly Prepared

■ **Please, I would like this dish _____.**

S'il vous plaît, j'aimerais ce plat _____.
* baked—au four
* boiled—bouilli
* broiled—grillé
* cold—froid
* fried—frît
* grilled—grillé
* hot—très chaud
* medium—à point
* poached—poché
* rare—saignant
* roasted—rôti
* sautéed—sauté
* steamed—à la vapeur
* well done—bien cuit
* with all visible fat trimmed before cooking—avec tout le gras retiré avant la cuisson

■ **Please, I would like it with/without _____.**

S'il vous plaît, je l'aimerais avec/sans _____.
* black pepper—poivre
* butter (unsalted)—beurre (sans sel)
* cayenne—poivre de cayenne
* cream—crème fraîche
* dressing—vinaigrette
* fresh milk—lait frais
* gravy—jus
* margarine—margarine
* saccharin—saccharine
* salt—sel

- sauce—sauce
- seasoning—assaisonnement
- skim milk—lait écrémé
- sugar—sucre
- sweetening—substance pour sucrer

# Possible Replies

■ **Mr./Ms./Waiter/Manager/Maitre D': Please point to your reply. Thank you.**

Monsieur/Madame, s'il vous plaît, indiquez-moi votre réponse. Merci.

■ **I understand but cannot help you.**

Je comprends mais ne puis vous aider.

■ **I can prepare it as you wish.**

Je peux le préparer comme vous le désirez.

■ **Wait, I'll ask the chef/the maitre d'.**

Attendez, je vais demander au chef/au maître d'hôtel.

■ **If you can wait a while, we can prepare it as you wish.**

Si vous attendez un peu, nous pouvons le préparer comme vous le désirez.

■ **With sufficient notice we can prepare a special dish for you. We need:**

En étant averti suffisament à l'avance, nous pouvons vous préparer un plat spécial. Il nous faut:
- 3 or 4 hours notice—3 ou 4 heures
- 24 hours notice—24 heures
- 2 days notice—2 jours

■ **Wait, I'll get someone who speaks English.**

Attendez, je vais chercher quelqu'un qui parle anglais.

# Appendix 4:
# Italian Food Preparation

## How to Make Sure Your Food Is Properly Prepared

■ **Please, I would like it _____.**
Per favore, lo vorrei _____.
- baked—al forno
- boiled—bollito
- broiled—alla griglia
- cold—freddo
- fried—fritto
- grilled—alla griglia
- hot—caldo
- medium—cotto al punto giusto
- poached (for eggs)—cotto in acqua bollente/ in camicia
- poached (for fish)—pesce lesso
- rare—al sangue/poco cotto
- roasted—arrosto
- sautéed—saltato/fritto in padella
- steamed—cotto a vapore
- well done—ben cotto
- with all visible fat trimmed before cooking—con tutto il grasso visibile tagliato prima della cottura

■ **Please, I would like it with/without _____.**
Per favore, lo vorrei con/senza _____.
- black pepper—pepe
- butter (unsalted)—burro dolce (senza sale)
- cream—panna
- dressing—condimento
- fresh milk—latte fresco
- gravy—sugo
- margarine—margarina

- red pepper—peperoncino
- saccharin—saccarina
- salt—sale
- sauce—salsa
- seasoning—condimento
- skim milk—scremato
- sugar—zucchero
- sweetening—dolcificante

# Possible Replies

**■ Please point to your reply. Thank you.**
Per favore indichi la Sua risposta. Grazie.

**■ I understand but cannot help you.**
Capisco ma non La posso aiutare.

**■ I can prepare it as you wish.**
Posso prepararlo come vuole Lei.

**■ Wait, I'll ask the chef/the maitre d'.**
Aspetti, chiederò allo chef/al maitre d'hotel.

**■ If you wait a while, we can prepare it as you wish.**
Se può aspettare un pò, possiamo prepararlo come vuole.

**■ With sufficient notice we can prepare a special dish for you. We need:**
Se ce lo fa sapere in anticipo, le possiamo preparare un piatto speciale. Abbiamo bisogno di saperlo:
- 3 or 4 hours notice—3 o 4 ore in anticipo
- 24 hours notice—24 ore in anticipo
- 2 days notice—2 giorni in anticipo

**■ Wait, I'll get someone who speaks English.**
Aspetti, vado a prendere qualcuno che parla Inglese.